Kindly Donated

by

Mr Lewis

TUBAL

INFERTILITY

Ivo A. Brosens MD PhD
Professor of Obstetrics and Gynaecology
Catholic University of Leuven
Leuven, Belgium

Alan G. Gordon MB BCh FRCS FRCOG
Consultant Gynaecologist
Princess Royal Hospital
Hull, UK

Foreword by:
Howard W. Jones Jr. MD FRCOG
Professor of Obstetrics and Gynecology
Eastern Virginia Medical School
Norfolk, Virginia, USA
and
Professor Emeritus of Obstetrics and
    Gynecology
Johns Hopkins University School of Medicine
Baltimore, Maryland, USA

T U B A L

INFERTILITY

J.B. Lippincott Company   PHILADELPHIA

Gower Medical Publishing   LONDON · NEW YORK

Distributed in UK and Continental Europe by:
Harper & Row Ltd
Middlesex House
34–42 Cleveland Street
London W1P 5FB
UK

Distributed in USA and Canada by:
J.B. Lippincott Company
East Washington Square
Philadelphia, PA 19105
USA

Distributed in Philippines/Guam, Middle East, Latin America and Africa by:
Harper & Row International
10 East 53rd Street
New York, NY 10022
USA

Distributed in Southeast Asia, Hong Kong, India and Pakistan by:
Harper & Row Publishers (Asia) Pte Ltd
37 Jalan Pemimpin 02–01
Singapore 2057

Distributed in Japan by:
Igaku Shoin Ltd
Tokyo International
P.O. Box 5063
Tokyo
Japan

Distributed in Australia and New Zealand by:
Harper & Row (Australasia) Pty Ltd
P.O. Box 226
Artarmon, N.S.W. 2064
Australia

Publisher:	Fiona Foley
Project Editor:	Lindy van den Berghe
Design & Illustration:	Balvir Koura
Line artists:	Marion Tasker
	Jenni Miller
Index:	Anita Reid
Production:	Seamus Murphy

Library of Congress Catalog Number: 89-80850
Library of Congress Cataloging Publication Data are available
British Library Cataloguing in Publication Data:
Brosens, Ivo
  Tubal infertility
  1. Women. Tubal infertility
  I. Title.   II. Gordon, Alan
  618.1'78

ISBN 0-397-44572-5 (Lippincott/Gower)

Originated in Singapore by Colourscan Overseas Co Pte Ltd
Typesetting by M to N Typesetters, London
Text set in Garamond; captions and figures set in News Gothic
Produced by Mandarin Offset. Printed in Hong Kong

FOREWORD

Anyone who accepts the responsibility to investigate and treat infertile couples needs to benefit from the studies and experience of Ivo Brosens and Alan Gordon. These workers have long investigated the tubal and peritoneal factors responsible for reproductive mischief and have clearly presented their new and novel findings in summary form in this lavishly illustrated book. Although experts have been called upon to write about six very specialized topics, the bulk of the work is out of the personal experience of the senior authors and therefore has the ring of authenticity which is so superior to a mere gleaning of the literature.

Thus, we hear first-hand of such new developments as the critical use of salpingoscopy to estimate the possible benefits of tubal surgery and to help assign patients to proper categories of therapy as well as the newer findings concerning incipient endometriosis with its critical implication for classifying this curious disease into endocrine-sensitive and endocrine-resistant forms.

Thus, this book has very practical information which translates into the best contemporary care for the female partners of those couples whose fertility is impaired by tubal or peritoneal factors.

Howard W. Jones Jr.
Norfolk, Virginia

PREFACE

In the last decade there have been major advances in the understanding and treatment of infertility due to disease of the fallopian tubes. A knowledge of the pathology of the tube and related disease of the peritoneum and ovary enables the clinician to utilize fully the modern diagnostic and therapeutic modalities essential for the correct treatment of the infertile woman.

In this new book we have drawn on our own clinical experience of infertility and have also brought together the work of some of the foremost authorities on the pathology, investigation and treatment of tubal disease. Microphotographs and clinical colour pictures have been used to enable both the postgraduate student and the established specialist to increase his/her knowledge and understanding of this fascinating subject.

The ultrastructure of the tubal mucosa has been studied by Dr Gloria Vasquez in Leuven and it is a great pleasure to include her work in the chapter in which the abnormal fallopian tube is discussed. It is impossible to separate disease of the fallopian tube from diseases of the ovary and pelvic peritoneum, so Dr Freddy Cornillie has contributed a chapter on the fine structure of the normal peritoneum and the peritoneum with endometriotic implants. We have attempted to put in perspective the relationship between peritoneal and ovarian endometriosis and infertility and have also introduced new concepts in the endoscopic treatment of ovarian endometriosis.

The diagnosis of tubal disease involves detailed examination of the whole genital tract by radiological and endoscopic methods. Dr Bruno van Herendael has added to our knowledge of the appearance of the internal tubal ostium in infertility. The accepted place of laparoscopy is discussed in detail and a new endoscopic technique, laparoscopic salpingoscopy, which has been developed in the past three years, is described.

We are pleased to acknowledge our debt to four of the foremost workers in the field of infertility who have contributed on their specialized subjects: Professor Willy Boeckx on tubal microsurgery, Dr Thierry Vancaillie on laparoscopic electrosurgery, Dr Dan C. Martin on laser surgery and Professor Ricardo Asch on new aspects of gamete intrafallopian transfer.

We would like to thank Dr Patrick Puttemans of the St-Elisabeth Hospital, Brussels who has been associated with the development of the salpingoscope and ovarioscope, Dr Margaret Leake of the University of Hull for her assistance with preliminary editing and Mr Luc de Simpelaere of the University Hospital, Leuven, who was responsible for much of the photography. Finally we would like to acknowledge our debt to Miss Balvir Koura for the design of this book and to express our appreciation of the constant support of the Project Editor, Dr Lindy van den Berghe, of Gower Medical Publishing.

Ivo Brosens
Alan Gordon
Leuven and Hull, 1989

CONTENTS

CONTRIBUTORS

Ricardo H. Asch MD
Professor of Obstetrics and Gynecology
University of California, Irvine
California, USA

Willy Boeckx MD PhD
Professor of Plastic Surgery
Catholic University of Leuven
Leuven, Belgium

Freddy Cornillie DSc
Research Fellow
Department of Obstetrics and Gynaecology
University Hospital Gasthuisberg
Leuven, Belgium

Bruno van Herendael MD
Head of Department of Reproductive Medicine
Jan Palfijn General Hospital
Antwerp, Belgium

Dan C. Martin MD
Clinical Assistant Professor
Department of Obstetrics and Gynecology
University of Tennessee
Memphis, Tennessee, USA

Thierry Vancaillie MD
Assistant Professor, Obstetrics and Gynecology
University of Texas
San Antonio, Texas, USA

1 THE NORMAL FALLOPIAN TUBE

1.1 History

1.2 Anatomy of the Fallopian Tube

1.3 Physiology of the Fallopian Tube

1.1 HISTORY

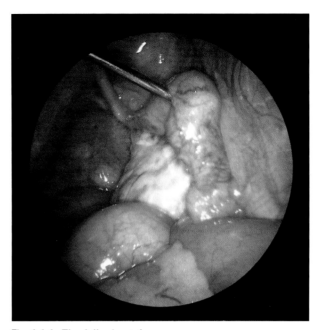

Fig. 1.1.1 The fallopian tube.
Laparoscopic view of the right fallopian tube, which has been
lifted with a probe so that the fimbriae can be inspected.

The first accurate description of the oviduct (Fig. 1.1.1)
was provided by Gabriele Falloppio in his 'Observa-
tiones Anatomicae' in 1561: 'This seminal duct originates from the cornua uteri, it is thin, very narrow, of
white colour, and looks like a nerve. After a short
distance it begins to broaden and to coil like a tendril,
winding its folds almost up to the end. There, having
becoming very broad, it shows an extremitas of the
nature of skin and colour of flesh, the utmost end
being very ragged and crushed like the fringe of worn
out clothes. Further, it has a great hole which is held
closed by the fimbriae which lap over each other.
However, if they spread out and dilate, they create a
kind of opening which looks like a flaring bell, the
brazen tube. Because the course of the seminal duct,
from its origin to its end resembles the shape of this
classical instrument, whether the curves are existing or
not, I named it the tuba uteri'.

In 1621 Fabricius described the secretory activity of
the 'upper part of the uterus' in the formation of the
avian egg, a function which was suggested much later
for the mammalian oviduct by Blundell in 1819, while
Dionis in 1724, pointed out the importance of tubal
motility, and compared it with the motility of the
intestine. He also provided an accurate description of
tubal pregnancy: 'if the egg is too big or if the diameter
of the tube fallopiana is too small, the egg stops and
can get no further, but shoots forth and takes root here
...' (Dionis, 1719). Riolanus the younger had previously
given the first description of ruptured tubal pregnancy
in 1604; this was later recognized by Moriceau, and
recorded in his 'Traité des Maladies des Femmes' in
1675.

The movement of the cilia was first recognized by
Purkinje and Valentin in 1834, who noticed that small
particles moved and rotated on the mucosal surface of
the rabbit oviduct. This observation helped to explain
the transport of the conceptus which previously had
been attributed to peristalsis of the tube: 'the forces
which lead the egg out of the ovary into and then
through the oviduct are in part the vibratory movement of the cilia of the epithelium of the infundibulum
and the mucosal membrane of the oviduct, and in part
the independent motion of the latter' (all cited by
Bodemer, 1968).

Interest in tubal disease developed during the second
half of the nineteenth century when the first reports on
tubal tumours appeared and genital tuberculosis was
described. *Neisseria gonorrhoeae* was discovered and
its association with salpingitis and infertility was
established. At the same time, the first operations for
ruptured tubal pregnancy and for other tubal pathology were reported.

The beginning of this century was marked by the
development of diagnostic procedures for tubal pathology with the introduction of hysterosalpingography,
tubal pertubation and laparoscopy. Results after conventional tubal surgery have varied widely and subsequent pregnancy rates of 0–50% have been reported.
During the last decade, the development and increasing
use of the operating microscope, encouraging an
atraumatic approach to surgery for infertility, has been
a significant advance in the repair of tubal damage. In
the 1980s, laparoscopic surgery with laser has achieved
equally good results and, when surgery has failed, *in
vitro* fertilization has provided hope to the woman
with tubal infertility.

1.2 ANATOMY OF THE FALLOPIAN TUBE

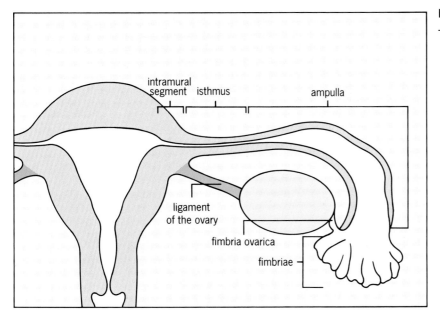

**Fig. 1.2.1 The fallopian tube
– a diagrammatic representation.**

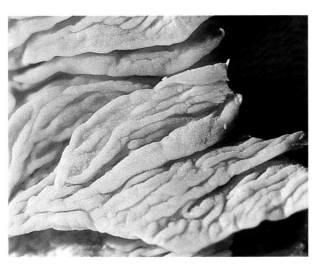

Fig. 1.2.2 The fimbriae.
Longitudinal section showing the concentration of mucosal folds towards the infundibulum.

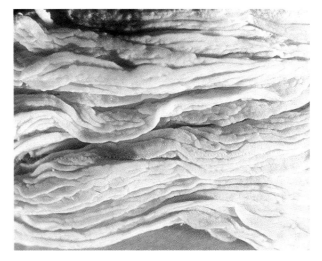

Fig. 1.2.3 The tubal ampulla.
The major mucosal folds and accessory folds can be clearly seen. The minor folds are hidden.

Tubal Segments

In women, as in many other mammalian species, four anatomical segments of the fallopian tube can be distinguished: the fimbriae, the ampulla, the isthmus and the intramural, or interstitial, segment (Fig. 1.2.1).

Fimbriae
The abdominal ostium of the tube is 1–1.5 cm in diameter and surrounded by fimbriae. In contrast to the richness of its folds (Fig. 1.2.2), this segment is poor in muscle fibres, with thin outer longitudinal and inner circular layers. The epithelium is densely ciliated, with ciliated cells which beat uniformly towards the uterus, representing more than 60% of the epithelial cell population in healthy fertile women.

Ampulla
The ampulla is the longest of the tubal segments, representing approximately 60% of its length. The lumen diameter varies from 1–2 mm at the isthmo-ampullary junction to 1 cm near the infundibulum. The mucosa contains 3–5 longitudinal major folds and between these are numerous smaller ones (Fig. 1.2.3).

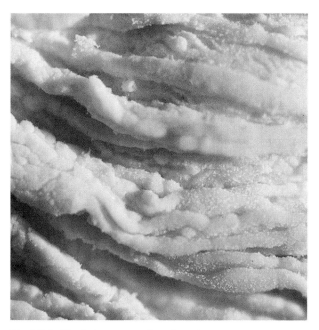

Fig. 1.2.4 The isthmo-ampullary junction.
The transition from the larger ampullary mucosal folds to the smaller isthmic folds is evident.

These folds have a rich network of blood vessels and lymphatics. The mucosa is densely ciliated with 40–60% of the total epithelial cells bearing cilia. These ciliated cells are numerous on the sides of the mucosal folds but their numbers decrease towards the apex. The ciliary beat throughout the ampulla is directed towards the uterus.

The muscle fibres are arranged in three layers comprising an outer longitudinal layer, a middle circular layer and an incomplete inner longitudinal layer.

Isthmus

The lumen of the isthmus averages 0.5 mm but can be as narrow as 0.1 mm, and the muscle layer is well developed, consisting of outer and inner longitudinal layers with a circular layer in between. The mucosal folds, usually 4–5 in number, are low and slightly rounded (Fig. 1.2.4). The ciliated cells comprise only 20–25% of the epithelial cells.

Intramural Segment

In the human, the intramural or interstitial segment of the uterine tube may have a straight, curved or convoluted course ending in a rounded or fish-mouthed opening at each cornual angle of the uterus. The muscular wall is composed of an inner and outer longitudinal layer with an intermediate circular layer arranged in a spiral fashion. The 2–3 tubal epithelial folds may extend into the uterine cavity or end a few mm from the ostium. The transition from intramural endosalpinx to cornual endometrium is marked by a transitional area with characteristic histological features. There is a marked decrease in the number of ciliated cells and the secretory cells tend to be flattened and assume a polygonal, elongated shape rather than their usual 'rounded-dome' appearance. The richness of the vascular supply and innervation suggests that this region acts as an adrenergic sphincter.

Histology of the Tubal Mucosa

The tubal mucosa consists of a simple columnar epithelium of ciliated and non-ciliated cells with a supporting tissue stroma that is rich in blood vessels and lymphatics. Three different cell types have been described in the tubal epithelium (Fig. 1.2.5).

Ciliated Cells

The ciliated cells are cuboidal, with finely granular cytoplasm and large central round or oval nuclei.

Secretory Cells

The secretory cells have a finely granular cytoplasm and their nuclei are wedge or oval-shaped, and dark. The position of the nuclei in the cells varies with the phase of the menstrual cycle (Fig. 1.2.6). During the follicular phase, the epithelium attains its greatest height and the secretory and ciliated cells are equally prominent, resulting in a regular luminal border. Late in the luteal phase, the cupolas of the secretory cells rupture, extruding cytoplasmic and nuclear material into the tubal lumen. Subsequently there is a marked irregularity of the border due to diminution in the height of the non-ciliated cells.

The 'peg' cells, or intercalary cells, look like slender pegs driven between the other cells. The nuclei commonly appear as wedge-like masses close to the basement membrane and are surrounded by a small amount of cytoplasm. 'Peg cells' are most numerous in the premenstrual and menstrual phases. Sometimes they cannot be distinguished from secretory cells, and these two types of cell are thought to represent different phases of the same life cycle.

Indifferent Cells

'Indifferent cells' form a small population of cells which lie along the base of the normal epithelium and cannot be identified by scanning electron microscopy because of their deep position. Their function is not fully understood but they may be the progenitors of the epithelial and stromal elements, or function in immunological defence.

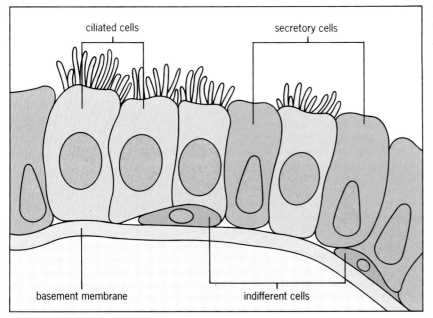

Fig. 1.2.5 The three different cell types found in tubal epithelium – a diagrammatic representation.

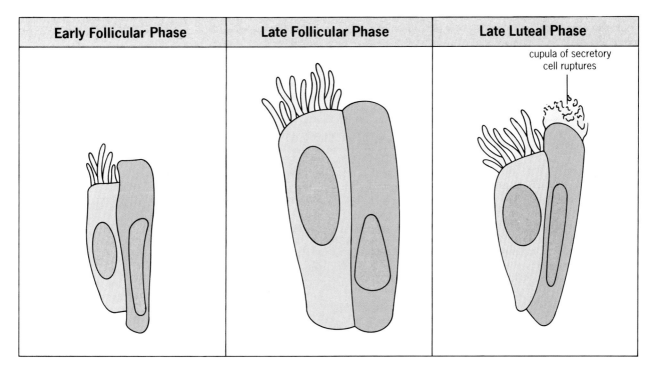

Fig. 1.2.6 Cyclical changes in the tubal epithelium.

Influence of the Menstrual Cycle

The specific changes in the morphology and distribution of the ciliated cells during the menstrual cycle are subject to debate. Both ciliated and secretory cells respond individually to ovarian steroid fluctuations, with responses such as an increase in size, and in the number of cytoplasmic granules and mitochondria, but the cyclical changes are less marked than those occurring in the endometrium. There is probably some renewal of ciliated cells, but mitotic activity has rarely been observed (Patek, 1973).

A number of investigators have found no evidence to show that ciliated cells undergo transformation into secretory cells in the human oviduct, or that they become desquamated, or that there is a cyclical variation in their distribution (Brosens & Vasquez, 1976).

However, Verhage *et al.* (1979), did find some deciliation in the late luteal phase particularly in the fimbriae. As this deciliation coincided with increased levels of progesterone in the peripheral plasma, they concluded that the induction and maintenance of a mature tubal epithelium is controlled by oestradiol, and antagonized by progesterone, despite the continued presence of oestradiol. Moreover, these investigators found that the process of cellular flattening and deciliation continued during pregnancy. Some degree of deciliation and reciliation in the fimbriae and distal ampulla has been reported during the menstrual cycle of Rhesus monkeys (Brenner, 1969).

Patek *et al.* (1972), failed to find any evidence of deciliation in the ampulla or fimbriae in the first 15 years after the menopause. However, in women 20–30 years after the menopause, they did find areas of flattened epithelium in the isthmus which lacked cilia and secretory activity, suggesting that tubal mucosal cells may be more refractory to ovarian steroids than those of the endometrium.

Although there is disagreement concerning the morphological changes in ciliated tubal cells, it is generally accepted that it is the individual cell rather than the tissue which undergoes cyclical changes.

Vascular Anatomy

The Arterial and Venous System

The blood supply of the fallopian tubes (Fig. 1.2.7) is derived from the uterine and ovarian arteries and varies not only between individuals, but also between the two sides of the pelvis; it is possible that only one of the arteries is sufficient to supply the whole length of the tube (Borrell & Fernstrom, 1953). The formation of an arcade of vessels in the mesosalpinx running parallel to the tube is an almost constant finding. The parietal arteries originate individually from the arcade. After following a tortuous subserous pathway towards the antimesenteric border of the tube and giving rise to numerous collaterals, they penetrate the muscularis and follow the different muscle layers until, on reaching the mucosa, they end in numerous capillaries (Gillet *et al.*, 1979).

The veins follow the arterial pathways. A venous plexus in the submucosa and another in the muscularis drain the capillary bed from the mucosa, submucosa and muscularis. The intratubal venous plexuses drain towards the external iliac vein.

The Lymphatic System

The lymphatic system of the fallopian tube consists of three subsystems: a mucosal system, an intramuscular

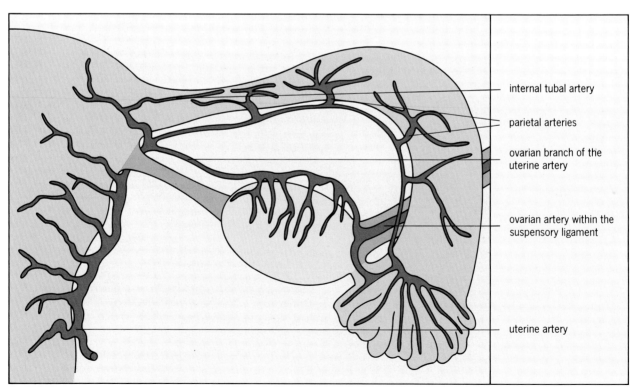

internal tubal artery

parietal arteries

ovarian branch of the uterine artery

ovarian artery within the suspensory ligament

uterine artery

Fig. 1.2.7 Blood supply of the fallopian tube.

system and a subserous system (Fig. 1.2.8).

The mucosal lymph capillaries are highly developed, particularly in the fimbriae and ampulla where they probably play a role in functions such as ovum pick-up, ovum transport and fertilization. These lymph capillaries drain into two plexuses located at the bases of the folds, which in turn drain into the intramuscular lymphatic system that develops with the onset of puberty and undergoes involutionary changes after the menopause.

The subserous lymphatic system collects lymph from both the intramuscular lymphatics and from others originating directly from the mucosal system. Finally, the lymphatic vessels enter the mesosalpinx and drain into the para-aortic and lumbar nodes. The lymphatic network of the fimbria ovarica drains directly into the mesosalpinx.

Innervation

The fallopian tube has both a sympathetic and para-sympathetic innervation. The sympathetic fibres originate from the 10th thoracic to the 2nd lumbar segment and end in the inferior mesenteric ganglion. The postganglionic fibres supply the isthmus and the proximal ampulla via the hypogastric plexus and the hypogastric nerve. Other sympathetic pre-ganglionic fibres which

originate from the 10th and 11th thoracic segments synapse in the coeliac, aortic and renal ganglia, the postganglionic fibres reaching the ovarian plexus and supplying the fimbriae and distal ampulla.

The 'long' adrenergic neurons originating in the inferior mesenteric ganglion and 'short' adrenergic neurons emanating from the cervico-vaginal ganglia close to the effector organ, supply the myosalpinx. In addition to their structural differences, these long and short neurons have different physiological actions (Black, 1974).

The distribution of sympathetic fibres is most dense in the isthmus and isthmo-ampullary junction, particularly in the circular muscle layer, but is sparse and located around blood vessels in the ampulla. α-receptors in the oviduct are stimulatory, while β-receptors are inhibitory. Adrenergic neuronal mechanisms seem to have a role in the mediation of the periovulatory changes in tubal contractility which occur in response to steroid hormone changes.

The less pronounced parasympathetic innervation is supplied in the proximal region by the pelvic nerve formed by fibres derived from the 2nd to 4th sacral segments, and in the distal region by the vagal nerve via the ovarian plexus.

The afferent neurons which carry pain sensation from the tube run with the fibres from the sympathetic autonomic system.

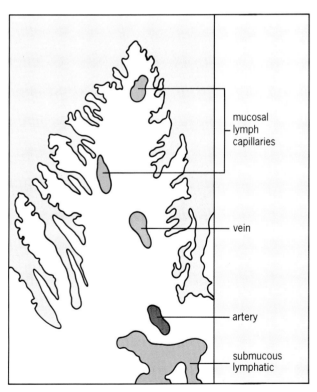

Fig. 1.2.8 Lymphatic drainage of the fallopian tube.

1.3 PHYSIOLOGY OF THE FALLOPIAN TUBE

The fallopian tube has the complex task of ensuring the transport of spermatozoa towards the ovary, and of ova towards the uterus. In addition, it supports the changes in the gametes which lead to fertilization, embryo cleavage and transport of the zygote towards the normal site of implantation in the uterine endometrium.

Ovum Pick-up

In some mammals, recovery of the oöcyte released from the follicle by the fimbriae is ensured by the presence of an ovarian bursa which encloses the ovarian surface and the fimbriae, permitting capture of the free oöcyte in the bursal cavity (Blandau, 1968). This bursa may be completely closed as in rats, or may have a small opening as in dogs. Alternatively, in other species such as the rabbit, the fimbriae remain in close contact with the ovary enclosing it completely at ovulation or, as in the human, nearly enclosing it, by the dual action of the fimbria ovarica and the ovarian mesentery. The fimbriae are directed to the site of ovulation by the muscular contractions of the mesosalpinx and tubo-ovarian ligaments (Fig. 1.3.1). The newly released oöcyte, contained within its sticky cumulus, attaches to the fimbrial cilia, and is swept from the surface of the ovary and propelled towards the tubal peritoneal ostium by the vigorous beating of the cilia (Odor & Blandau, 1973). Most authors agree that this is the main mechanism by which ova enter the fallopian tube. However, the following experimental and clinical observations have suggested other mechanisms.

1. Ova may enter fallopian tubes which have no direct contact with the surface of the ovary, as in women with one ovary and a contralateral fallopian tube, or they may enter the tube on the side opposite the corpus luteum. The frequency with which contralateral ovum pick-up occurs in normal circumstances is unknown. The most probable explanation of this is ovum pick-up from the cul-de-sac or from peritoneal fluid currents which carry the egg and eventually approximate it to the fimbriae. Pick-up from the pouch of Douglas fluid is the probable pathway of ova entering tubal fistulae proximal to a ligated tubal segment (Metz, 1977) and by fertilized ova which implant in accessory tubes or in an abnormally located oviduct far from the ovulation surface.

2. Westman's studies in 1937 suggested that ova could be 'sucked' into the oviducts by tubal peristaltic activity. This was supported by a report on negative pressure caused by tubal contractions (Maia & Coutinho, 1970). However, it has been shown that oviducts ligated at the base of the fimbriae are still able to pick up ova efficiently (Clewe & Mastroianni, 1958). Similarly, when the contractility of an oviduct is blocked by propanolol, ovum pick-up and transport can still occur (Halbert & Patton, 1976).

3. Ova enter the fallopian tubes in women with the Immotile Cilia Syndrome, therefore more than one mechanism must be essential for optimum ovum pick-up.

4. Experimental work in rabbits has suggested that the fimbriae are not essential to fertility (Beyth & Winston,

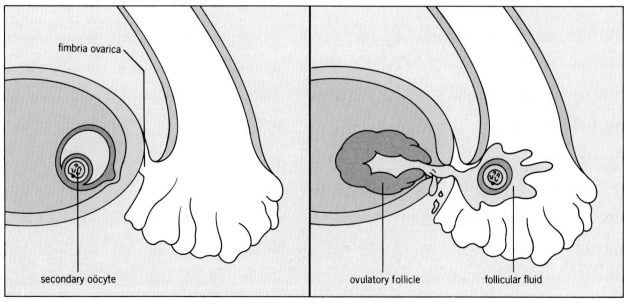

Fig. 1.3.1a & b Ovulation and ovum pick-up.
a The fimbriae are directed to the site of ovulation.

b The oöcyte attaches to the fimbrial cilia.

1981), though only 50% of women with patent oviducts achieve a pregnancy after reversal of fimbriectomy sterilization.

Ovum Transport

During its passage towards the uterus the ovum is retained in the ampulla for longer than in the rest of the tube and, while in this segment, ovum maturation, fertilization and early embryo cleavage occur. In women, both fertilized and unfertilized ova remain in the ampulla for approximately 72 hours (Croxatto *et al.*, 1972) which is a similar period of time to that reported in other primates (Eddy *et al.*, 1975).

The ciliary beat and the peristaltic and segmental contraction of the muscle wall are involved in transporting the ovum through the ampulla. It has been postulated that in order to effect cilial propulsion, the ovum should be in contact with the luminal wall, and touching the ciliated sides of the closely opposed folds of the ampulla.

In the isthmus, muscular contractions are mainly responsible for ovum transport. Retention at the isthmo-ampullary junction is common in most mammals including humans, although it is not as marked in women as in rabbits. This retention could result from the interaction of the cilia beating towards the uterus, the tubal fluid currents flowing towards the ovary, and both peristaltic and segmental muscular contraction. The secretory activity of the isthmus is maximal at ovulation when a highly viscous and tenacious mucus is produced which fills the lumen and blocks ovum passage towards this segment (Jansen, 1978). Isthmic subserosal oedema due to the dilatation of the venous system in response to oestrogens could contribute to this closure as suggested by work in rabbits.

It is generally agreed that muscular contractions of the tube play an important role in both ovum retention at the isthmo-ampullary junction and further transport of the ovum towards the uterus. Study of the contractility of the oviductal smooth muscle has, however, proved difficult.

Sperm Transport and Activation

In women, spermatozoa may be found in the oviduct a few minutes after their deposition in the vagina (Settlage *et al.*, 1973). During their passage through the uterus and into the oviduct their own motility is assisted by uterine peristaltic contractions stimulated by oxytocin and both uterine and seminal prostaglandins. Only a small proportion of the ejaculated spermatozoa enter the oviduct with approximately 200 reaching the ampulla which is the site of fertilization (Ahlgreen,

1975). As these spermatozoa have the greatest motility, and, like those which eventually reach the peritoneal cavity, are morphologically normal, a quantitative and a qualitative control mechanism must exist.

Both the utero-tubal junction and the isthmus appear to act as functional barriers and filters. The utero-tubal junction relaxes, enabling spermatozoa to enter the oviduct. This relaxation results from the response of the musculature to progesterone, prostaglandins, oxytocin, adrenaline and other influences. In the isthmus, muscular peristaltic contractions could control the release of sperm towards the ampulla. Also, the isthmic secretion protects the spermatozoa from the beating of the ciliary shafts towards the uterus. Thus, in humans, the cilia do not appear to participate in sperm transport. In other mammals such as rabbits and pigs, however, two-way ciliary transport currents and the movement of sperm may be assisted by cilia beating towards the ovary.

Motile sperm may be found in the ampulla and peritoneal cavity as late as 80–85 hours after coitus. Although some authors claim that the ability of spermatozoa to fertilize the ovum may be restricted to only half their motile life, others claim that the spermatozoa have this ability for a much longer period.

In order to fertilize an oöcyte, the spermatozoa need to undergo a phenomenon called capacitation (Austin, 1951; Chang, 1951). This involves the gradual removal of the plasma membrane coatings from the acrosomal region of the spermatozoa by lytic agents and is normally achieved during the passage of the sperm through the genital tract; both the tubal and uterine environments seem to be important (Fig. 1.3.2). The process may also be completed in the cervical canal and can be induced *in vitro* with relative ease by exposure to a well defined culture medium. Once completed, capacitation permits sperm to incorporate calcium ions which are required to initiate the acrosome reaction (Bedford, 1970). Whereas morphological studies have failed to show the specific changes of the sperm membranes occurring due to capacitation, the acrosome reaction is well documented by ultrastructural studies (Van Blerkom & Motta, 1979).

Embryo Transport

With the initiation of cleavage, the cytoplasm of the embryo begins its successive division into blastomeres. This is accompanied by major changes in the cytoplasm and in the synthesis of macromolecules, but with no increase in the diameter of the embryo. Up to the 8 or 16 cell stage, cleavage is regular, resulting in equally sized blastomeres. From this stage onwards, the outer cells lose their distinct cell outlines, develop desmosomes and later, tight junctions, therefore forming a compact outer cell layer which surrounds an inner cell mass.

The embryo begins to divide in the ampulla and cleavage continues during its passage towards the uterus. Human embryos have been found to enter the uterus as early as the 8 and 12 cell stages (Fig. 1.3.3).

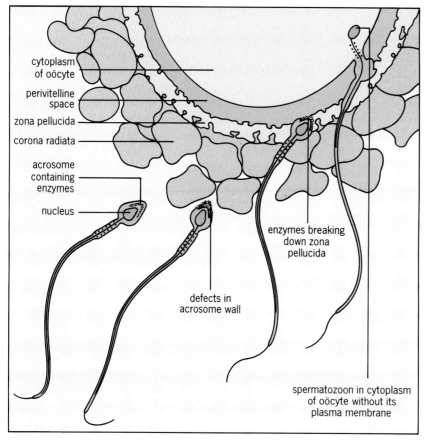

Fig. 1.3.2 Capacitation of a spermatozoon and its subsequent penetration of an oöcyte.
Capacitation involves the gradual removal of the plasma membrane coatings from the acrosomal region of the spermatozoon so that enzymes can be released to break down the zona pellucida.

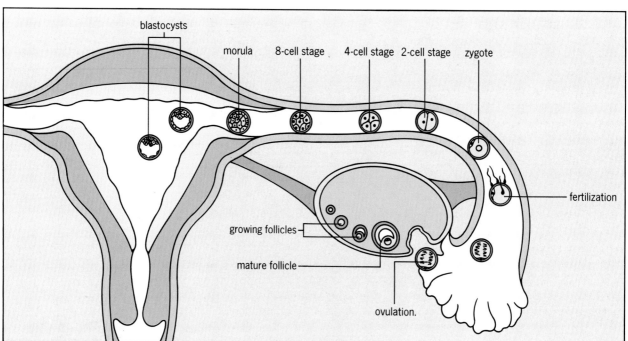

Fig. 1.3.3 Oöcyte release, fertilization, transport and division into blastomeres.

REFERENCES

Ahlgreen, M. (1975) Sperm transport to and survival in the human fallopian tube. *Gynecological Investigation*, **6**, 206–214.

Austin, C.R. (1951) Activation and correlation between male and female elements in fertilization. *Nature*, **168**, 558–559.

Bedford, J.M. (1970) Sperm capacitation and fertilization in mammals. *Biology of Reproduction* (Suppl.), **2**, 128–158.

Beyth, Y. & Winston, R.M.L. (1981) Ovum capture and fertility following microsurgical fimbriectomy in the rabbit. *Fertility and Sterility*, **35**, 464–466.

Black, D.L. (1974) Neuronal control of oviduct musculature. In: *The Oviduct and its Functions*. Edited by A.D. Johnson & C.W. Foley, p.65. London: Academic Press.

Blandau, R.J. (1968) Gamete transport – comparative aspects. In: *The Mammalian Oviduct*. Edited by E.S.E. Hafez & R.J. Blandau, pp.129–162. Chicago: The University of Chicago Press.

Bodemer, C.W. (1968) History of the mammalian oviduct. In: *The Mammalian Oviduct*. Edited by E.S.E. Hafez & R.J. Blandau, pp.3–26. Chicago: The University of Chicago Press.

Borrell, U. & Fernstrom, I. (1953) The adnexal branches of the uterine artery. An arteriographic study in humans. *Acta Radiologica*, **40**, 561–582.

Brenner, R.M. (1969) Renewal of oviduct cilia during the menstrual cycle of the Rhesus monkey. *Fertility and Sterility*, **20**, 599–611.

Brosens, I.A. & Vasquez, G. (1976) Fimbrial microbiopsy. *Journal of Reproductive Medicine*, **16**, 171–178.

Chang, M.C. (1951) Fertilizing capacity of spermatozoa deposited in the fallopian tubes. *Nature*, **168**, 697–698.

Clewe, T.H. & Mastroianni, L.Jr. (1958) Mechanism of ovum pickup: I. Functional capacity of rabbit oviducts ligated near the fimbriae. *Fertility and Sterility*, **9**, 13–17.

Croxatto, F.N., Carrillo, D. & Fabres, C. (1972) Studies on the duration of egg transport in the human oviduct. I. The time interval between ovulation and egg recovery from the uterus in normal women. *Fertility and Sterility*, **23**, 447–458.

Eddy, C.A., Garcia, R.G., Kraemer, D.C. & Pauerstein, C.J. (1975) Detailed time-course of ovum transport in the Rhesus monkey (*Macaca mulatta*). *Biology of Reproduction*, **13**, 363–369.

Gillett, J.Y., Maillet, R. & Gautier, C. (1979) Anatomie descriptive et microvascularization de la trompe de fallope. In: *Oviducte et Fertilite*. Edited by I.A. Brosens, I.M. Cognat, A. Constantin & M. Thibier, pp.1–15. Paris: Masson.

Halbert, S.A. & Patton, D.L. (1976) Egg transport in the rabbit oviduct: the roles of cilia and muscle. *Science*, **191**, 1052–1053.

Jansen, R.P.S. (1978) Fallopian tube isthmic mucus and ovum transport. *Science*, **201**, 349–351.

Maia, H. & Coutinho, E.M. (1970) Peristalsis and antiperistalsis of the human fallopian tube during the menstrual cycle. *Biology of Reproduction*, **2**, 305–314.

Metz, K.G.P. (1977) Failures following fimbriectomy. *Fertility and Sterility*, **28**, 66–71.

Odor, D.L. & Blandau, R.J. (1973) Egg transport over the fimbrial surface of the rabbit oviduct under experimental conditions. *Fertility and Sterility*, **24**, 292–300.

Patek, E. (1973) Scanning electron microscopic observations on the ciliogenesis of the infundibulum of the human fetal and adult fallopian tube epithelium. *Fertility and Sterility*, **24**, 819.

Patek, E., Nilsson, J. & Johannison, E. (1972) Scanning electron microscopic study of the human fallopian tube. Report II. Fetal life, reproductive life and postmenopause. *Fertility and Sterility*, **23**, 719–733.

Settlage, D.F., Motoshima, M. & Tredway, D. (1973) Sperm transport from the external cervical os to the fallopian tubes in women: a time and quantitation study. *Fertility and Sterility*, **24**, 655–661.

Van Blerkom, J. & Motta, P. (1979) *The Cellular Basis of Mammalian Reproduction*, pp.136–138. Munich: Urband and Schwarzenberg.

Verhage, H.G., Bareither, M.L., Jaffe, R.C. & Akbar, M. (1979) Cyclic changes in ciliation, secretion and cell height of the oviductal epithelium in women. *American Journal of Anatomy*, **156**, 505–522.

Westman, A. (1937) Investigations into the transit of ova in man. *Journal of Obstetrics and Gynaecology of the British Empire*, **44**, 821–838.

2 THE ABNORMAL FALLOPIAN TUBE

2.1 The Sequelae of Pelvic Inflammatory Disease

2.2 Hydrosalpinx

2.3 Proximal Tubal Pathology

2.4 Tuberculosis

2.5 Tubal Pregnancy

2.6 Poststerilization

2.7 Congenital Tubal Anomalies

2.1   THE SEQUELAE OF PELVIC INFLAMMATORY DISEASE

Aetiology of Pelvic Inflammatory Disease

Damage resulting from infection is the commonest cause of tubal infertility. The aetiology of salpingitis has changed over the years; Westman (1950) found that tuberculosis, gonorrhoea, infection resulting from abortion and childbirth, and infections of unknown origin occurred with equal frequency in women with pelvic inflammatory disease (PID). More recent studies in developed countries have shown however that the most common causes are sexually transmitted 'non-specific' infection, and post-abortion and post-partum salpingitis (Westrom, 1980). Current studies have demonstrated *Chlamydia trachomatis* in a significant percentage of tubes during operations for the sequelae of pelvic inflammatory disease, and in Scandinavia this has become the commonest sexually transmitted organism and the most frequent cause of salpingitis. Moreover salpingitis occurs more commonly in younger women (Fig. 2.1.1).

Other organisms may also be implicated. These include *Mycoplasma hominis* which has occasionally been isolated from inflamed tubes and peritoneal exudate, and *Ureaplasma urealyticum*, group A streptococci and *Haemophilus influenzae*, which are uncommonly associated with acute salpingitis.

There is no unanimous opinion as to which microorganisms are most important in the aetiology of infection of the fallopian tubes, and differences in population and isolation techniques may be major factors influencing the results of the studies performed so far. More than one species may be implicated in the same infective episode, and a polymicrobial aetiology seems to be generally accepted. It is possible that anaerobic organisms may secondarily invade and further damage a fallopian tube primarily infected by gonococci or chlamydiae (Sweet *et al.*, 1979).

Salpingitis may present in an acute or chronic form, or as an acute exacerbation of a chronic infection. Both gonococci and chlamydiae ascend from the lower genital tract via the mucosal surfaces of the endocervix and endometrium to the endosalpinx. These microorganisms cause epithelial damage with loss of ciliated cells, and produce an inflammatory exudate which may

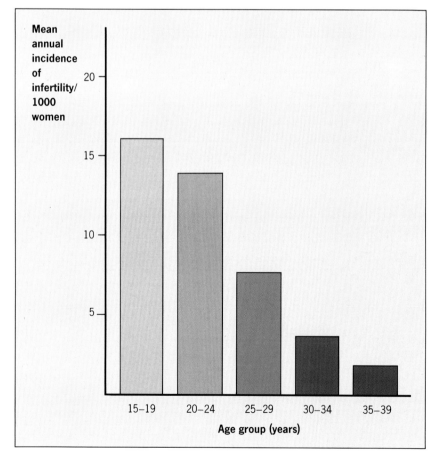

Fig. 2.1.1 Histogram showing the mean annual incidence of first episodes of salpingitis in the city of Lund between 1975 and 1979.

Based on data of Westrom, 1980.

cause adhesions between the mucosal folds. Strepto-cocci, staphylococci and Gram negative bacteria, which mainly cause puerperal, post-abortal and traumatic infections, probably reach the tubes via the lymphatic and vascular channels. It is probable that mycoplasmas also follow these pathways. The inflammatory process has been thought to affect the parametrium and tubal wall without damaging the endosalpinx. However, experimental intratubal inoculation of *Escherichia coli* in rabbits produces damage to both ciliated and non-ciliated cells, the damage being directly proportional to the dose of bacteria injected. The injury appears to be caused mainly by the endotoxins liberated from the cell walls of the bacteria (Laufer *et al.*, 1984).

Salpingitis can also occur as a result of adjacent or distant inflammatory processes and may be associated with infection in the bowel, such as appendicitis or diverticulitis. Although perisalpingeal involvement is the usual result of these conditions, tubal occlusion may occur secondarily to the neighbouring peritoneal reaction. Pre-pubertal salpingitis, although rare, is frequently associated with appendicular septic foci. Theoretically, haematogenous dissemination of an infection from any source may cause salpingitis as exemplified by the occurrence of pneumococcal sal-pingitis in children (Woodruff & Pauerstein, 1969). Salpingitis may also be caused by irritants or drugs introduced during uterine insufflation or surgery.

Sequelae of Salpingitis

The sequelae of salpingitis depend on the degree of tubal damage caused by the acute infective process, as only minor degrees of scarring result from complete resolution of mild inflammation. The obstructive con-sequences are generally accepted to be the principal cause of tubal infertility. However, Woodruff and Pauerstein (1969) believe that, in their cases, the extent of peritubal and periovarian adhesion is the primary determinant of tubal blockage and that intratubal pathology is of secondary importance. Studies on laparoscopically-confirmed salpingitis have shown that, with prompt diagnosis and treatment before the development of adnexal swelling, and in the absence of repeated infections, tubal patency and morphology is unlikely to be impaired (Jacobson & Westrom, 1969). Infertility occurs in 13% of patients who have had a single infection, but this incidence increases to 35% after two episodes and 75% after three or more infec-tions (Westrom, 1975; Fig. 2.1.2).

Pelvic inflammatory disease is the commonest cause of the tubal lesions responsible for ectopic pregnancy. In patients who have had conservative treatment for acute salpingitis, the risk of ectopic pregnancy is 1 in 24, whereas in healthy subjects it is 1 in 123. For women with intra-uterine contraceptive devices (IUCDs) however, the risk of ectopic pregnancy is 3–5 times higher than that of non-IUCD users. This risk is even higher in women with IUCDs who are also nulliparous or under 25 years of age (Westrom *et al.*, 1976). The high risk of tubal pregnancy among IUCD users may be related to their association with infection (Tatum & Schmidt, 1977).

The effect of IUCDs on the development of pelvic inflammatory disease seems to persist for several months after removal. Although the mechanism where-by these devices facilitate the spread of infection is not understood, there is evidence that the introduction of an IUCD causes bacterial contamination of the uterine cavity. Other factors in the infective process are the ascent of organisms from the lower genital tract along the attached tails and the muscular contractions of the uterus after insertion. This last hypothesis is supported by the observed increased risk of infection after a recent insertion or re-insertion. Most authors also report an increased risk of infection with prolonged use.

Whatever its aetiology, the sequelae of salpingitis which damages the distal portions of the fallopian tubes include hydrosalpinx, pyosalpinx, fimbrial partial

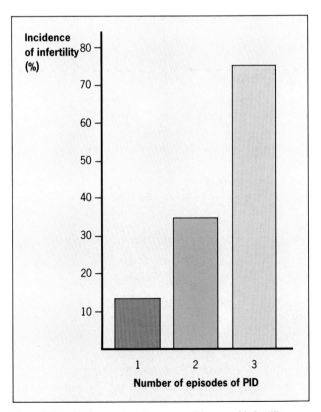

Fig. 2.1.2 Histogram showing the incidence of infertility after 1, 2 and 3 episodes of pelvic inflammatory disease. Based on data of Westrom, 1975.

obstruction without hydrosalpinx formation, and interstitial salpingitis. When the proximal segments of the tube are principally involved, the end-results include isthmic and cornual stenosis or blockage. Finally, the sequelae may involve the whole tube resulting in proximally blocked tubes with distal hydrosalpinges (Fig. 2.1.3). It is possible that salpingitis isthmica nodosa and haematosalpinx are also sequelae of pelvic inflammatory disease affecting the fallopian tubes.

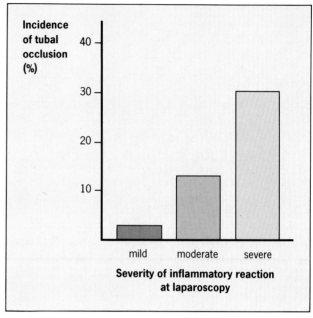

Fig. 2.1.3 Histogram showing the incidence of tubal occlusion associated with different degrees of inflammatory reaction at laparoscopy.
Based on data of Westrom and Mardh, 1977.

2.2 HYDROSALPINX

Hydrosalpinx caused by distal tubal blockage is a major cause of infertility.

Pathogenesis

In hydrosalpinx there is distal blockage and dilatation of the fallopian tube which is filled with clear, sterile, serous fluid. The aetiology of the condition is controversial.
1. Several authors believe that hydrosalpinx is the end-result of pyosalpinx where the infective process has been inactive for a long time (Woodruff & Pauerstein, 1969).
2. Alternatively, hydrosalpinx may be the primary lesion; in this case, pyosalpinx would occur secondarily to infection in it (Park, 1978).
3. A third theory is that there is an abnormality in the muscular wall of the tube and that hydrosalpinx is not a result of infection (Drapier et al., 1979).

The reason why dilatation can occur when only the distal end of the tube is blocked is not fully understood. Formation of a hydrosalpinx seems to depend on the rheological resistance induced by the narrow and frequently tortuous lumen of the intramural segment of the fallopian tube. Once the tube becomes distended by fluid its muscular contractions may not be strong enough to empty the lumen.

Gross Pathology

There are two classically recognized appearances of hydrosalpinx.
1. Hydrosalpinx simplex, in which the tube is dilated but there are no adhesions between the mucosal folds and thus the lumen is single.
2. Hydrosalpinx follicularis, in which the tubal lumen is divided into locules by mucosal folds which have agglutinated or adhered together forming compartments or pseudoglandular spaces.

At laparotomy or laparoscopy, a hydrosalpinx is seen to have either thin or thick walls. In thin-walled hydrosalpinx (Fig. 2.2.1), the fallopian tube is grossly distended by copious straw-coloured fluid which makes it appear translucent, whereas in thick-walled hydrosalpinx the wall is fibrous (Fig. 2.2.2), and the lumen is smaller and contains little fluid. In both types the terminal part of the tube is totally blocked and the fimbriae are obscured. The distinction between thin-walled and thick-walled hydrosalpinx is important; not only do their morphological and histological features differ, but also the pregnancy rate after tubal microsurgery is much lower for thick-walled than for thin-walled hydrosalpinx (Fig. 2.2.3).

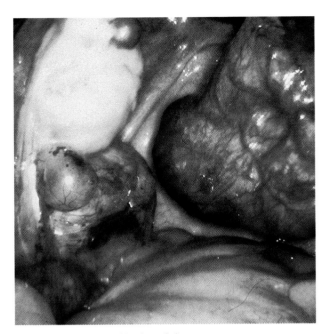

Fig. 2.2.1 Thin-walled hydrosalpinx.
The tube is markedly distended and the intrafallopian fluid can be seen through the semitransparent tubal wall. (Courtesy of Professor Kurt Semm.)

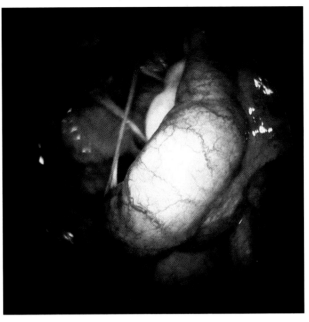

Fig. 2.2.2 Thick-walled hydrosalpinx.
Tubal distension is less marked than in thin-walled hydrosalpinx, and the intraluminal fluid cannot be seen.

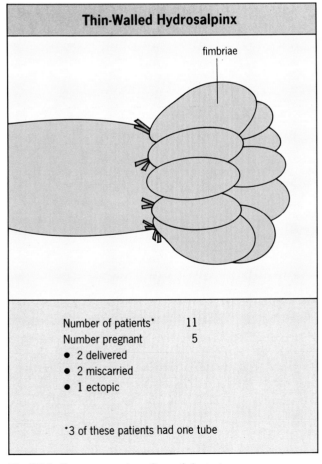

Thin-Walled Hydrosalpinx

fimbriae

Number of patients*   11
Number pregnant   5
● 2 delivered
● 2 miscarried
● 1 ectopic

*3 of these patients had one tube

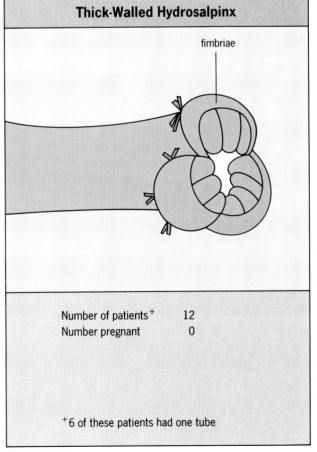

Thick-Walled Hydrosalpinx

fimbriae

Number of patients+   12
Number pregnant   0

+6 of these patients had one tube

Fig. 2.2.3 Pregnancy rates after salpingostomy.
The pregnancy rate after salpingostomy for thick-walled hydrosalpinx is much lower than after surgery for thin-walled hydrosalpinx.

Histopathology

Thin-Walled Hydrosalpinx

The mucosal surface of a thin-walled hydrosalpinx is smooth with flattened and sometimes markedly atrophied folds (Fig. 2.2.4a) which are often far apart and not parallel. This contrasts with the prominent, parallel and well opposed folds of the normal ampulla. There may be breaks in the continuity of the folds and adhesions between them, although the latter feature is more prominent in thick-walled hydrosalpinx. The formation of pseudoglandular spaces, which occurs in approximately 33% of cases, is less common than in thick-walled hydrosalpinx.

In the flattened areas, the epithelial cells are commonly desquamated (Fig. 2.2.4b), but this is less

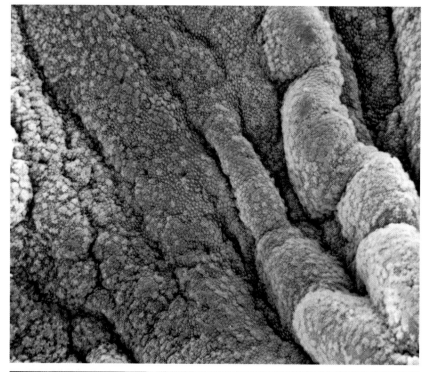

Fig. 2.2.4a–d Thin-walled hydrosalpinx.
a Scanning electronmicrograph (SEM) showing the flattened surface and the short, low mucosal folds (×180).

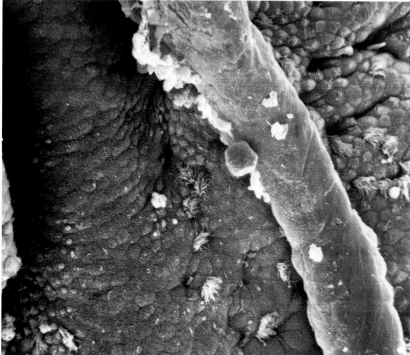

b SEM showing that the flattened mucosal folds are widely separated, and the extensive desquamation and deciliation of the mucosa (×230).

pronounced in areas where the folds are retained. There are also abnormalities of the cilia, which are significantly reduced in number and cover only a small part of the mucosal surface (Fig. 2.2.4c). In very distended tubes, non-ciliated cells are often stretched, polygonal or elongated with few microvilli or other surface abnormalities of the mucosal membrane (Fig. 2.2.4d). In the folded areas, the epithelial cells retain their columnar height, but where the mucosa is flattened, they become cuboidal. There may also be signs of cellular necrosis with condensed nuclear chromatin. The presence of lymphocytes and plasma cells indicates chronic inflammation, but this is usually confined to the stroma. Invaginations of the epithelium are often seen but do not reach the myosalpinx, which is thin and loses its differentiation into layers.

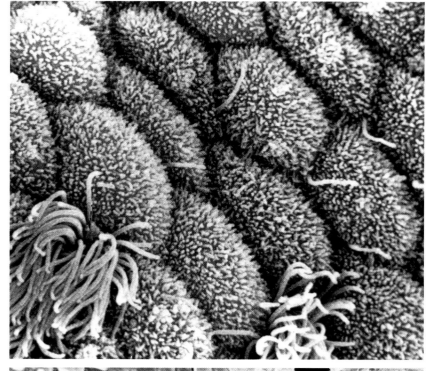

c SEM showing the non-ciliated cells with numerous microvilli. Occasional cells have a single villus (×4500).

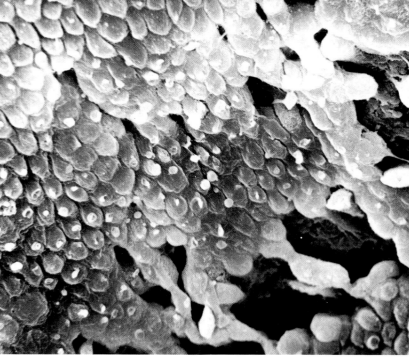

d SEM showing polygonal ciliated mucosal cells and epithelial desquamation (×500).

Thick-Walled Hydrosalpinx

Thick-walled hydrosalpinx is characterized either by a generalized agglutination of the folds (Fig. 2.2.5a), giving the mucosa a 'honeycomb' appearance due to the numerous pseudoglandular spaces (Fig. 2.2.5b), or by extreme atrophy of the folds. Deciliation is more variable and less uniform than in thin-walled hydrosalpinx. Desquamation of cells is also less common but is a prominent feature of the distended areas where the epithelial cells are low and cuboidal. Common abnormalities of the cilia include megacilia, cilia which are long and thin, and cilia with localized swollen areas

(Fig. 2.2.5c). The secretory cells are pleomorphic and the microvilli may be thick, fine or absent. Cupuloid or flat surface membranes and secretory blebs are present with varying frequency. One of the outstanding features is that totally different patterns of epithelial abnormalities may be found in neighbouring areas.

The stroma of a thick-walled hydrosalpinx contains epithelial invaginations with inflammatory cell infiltration. Lymphocytes, plasma cells and macrophages are clustered around the blood vessels, and occasionally extend to the myosalpinx and serosa. In addition there is usually extensive fibrosis of the tubal wall.

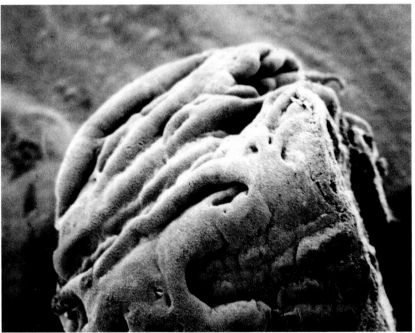

Fig. 2.2.5a–c Thick-walled hydrosalpinx.
a SEM showing extensive agglutination of the mucosa and adhesions between the folds (×100).

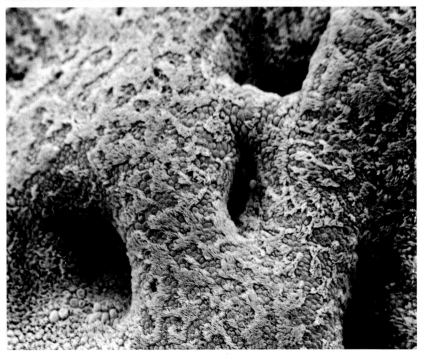

b SEM showing agglutination between the folds producing a 'honeycomb' appearance and forming pseudoglandular spaces (×250).

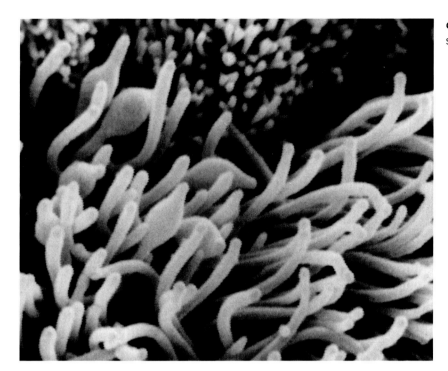

c SEM showing the cilia with thickened
segments near their tips (×11,500).

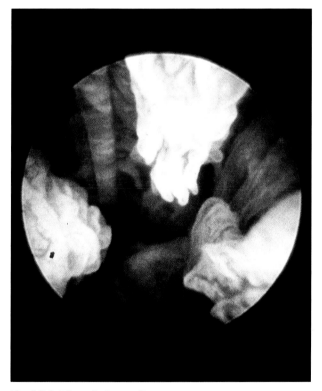

Fig. 2.2.6 The tubal ampulla.
Salpingoscopic view showing normal mucosa comprising 5–6
major folds arranged radially and running longitudinally.
Secondary folds arise from the sides of the major folds and the
minor folds lie between them.

Classification

In hydrosalpinx, examination of the tubes by laparoscopy reveals four different degrees of occlusion.
1. Patent tubes with conglutination or phimosis of the fimbrial folds.
2. Complete distal occlusion, but the diameter of the ampulla remains normal.
3. Complete distal occlusion, with the ampulla dilated to a diameter of 15–25 mm.
4. Complete distal occlusion, with the ampulla distended to a diameter of more than 25 mm – this is the classical hydrosalpinx simplex.

Salpingoscopy performed at the time of tubal microsurgery or at laparoscopy in patients with hydrosalpinx has led to the recognition of the following five different mucosal fold patterns:
1. Normal mucosal folds (Fig. 2.2.6).
2. The major and minor folds are preserved but wider apart than normal and there is a variable degree of flattening (Fig. 2.2.7a).
3. The major and minor folds are preserved, but there are focal lesions such as agglutination or adhesions (Figs 2.2.7b & 2.2.7c).
4. Extensive lesions of both major and minor folds, such as adhesions, stricture of the lumen and formation of pseudospaces (Fig. 2.2.7d).
5. The pattern of the folds is completely lost, the lumen is dilated and its walls appear rigid (Fig. 2.2.7e).

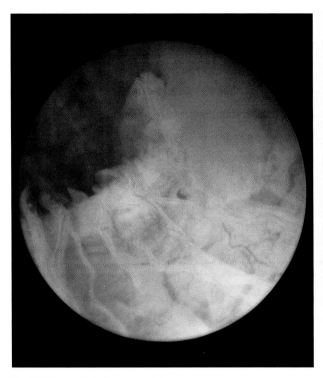

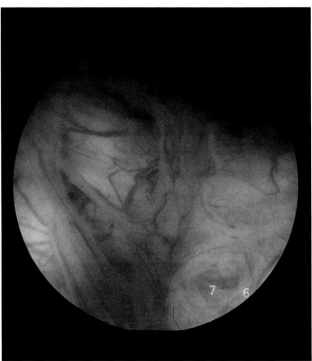

Fig. 2.2.7a–e Tubal mucosal damage.
a Grade 1. The major and minor folds are preserved with slight flattening.

b Grade 2. The folds are focally agglutinated.

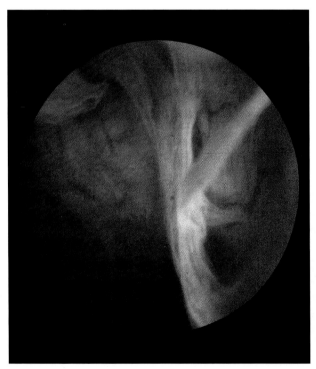

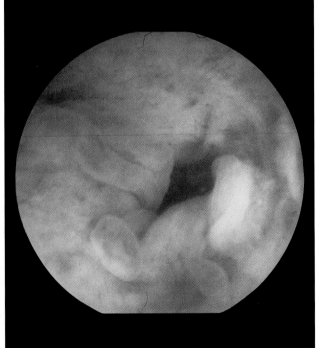

c Grade 2. Focal adhesions are evident between the mucosal folds.

d Grade 3. There are extensive adhesions with formation of pseudospaces.

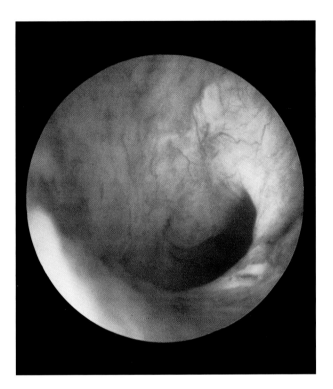

e Grade 4. The tube is rigid and the normal fold pattern is lost.

Discussion

Hydrosalpinx formation is frequently associated with extensive lesions of the mucosa. The cilia may be completely absent, agglutinated or adherent to each other, or they may be abnormal and disorganized. This could partly explain the failure of women with hydrosalpinx to conceive despite the patency of their tubes as, although the cilia are motile, their movements are incoordinate. Motile cilia are not, however, essential for conception; women with Kartagener's syndrome are known to have borne children, although their overall fertility is not recorded. Patients with the Kartagener triad have intact tubal musculature, presumably normal tubal secretions and a ciliated mucosal surface, but the cilia are non-motile. Perhaps even non-motile cilia may play a passive role in gamete transport by acting as a surface over which the egg can travel more easily than

over non-ciliated cells. Thus the situation in Kartagener's syndrome differs from that in patients with hydrosalpinx when much of the epithelial surface is devoid of cilia.

Restoration of tubal patency may partly improve the quality of the mucosa. Some of the mucosal damage, such as distension of the lumen, flattening of the folds, deciliation and even loss of epithelial cells may be secondary to stretching of the tubal wall. This situation is comparable to that in experimentally-produced hydrosalpinx in rabbits, where recovery of the mucosal lesions has been observed following salpingostomy and release of the mucosa from the pressure effects of the hydrosalpinx (Vasquez *et al.*, 1984). Whilst recovery of the ciliated cells can occur after patency is restored, it is likely that mucosal damage such as agglutination, adhesion formation and loss of folds, is irreversible.

2.3 PROXIMAL TUBAL PATHOLOGY

Proximal lesions of the fallopian tube occur less often than lesions of the distal end. Apart from surgical division of the tube, there are however a number of conditions affecting the intramural segment and the isthmus, which can cause infertility without necessarily producing complete obstruction of the lumen. The most common of these are obliterative fibrosis, salpingitis isthmica nodosa, chronic tubal inflammation and endometriosis. Less frequent causes are tubocornual polypi, tuberculosis and the remnants of a chronic tubal pregnancy. The results of surgical treatment depend on the nature and extent of the lesion. Patients with localized fibrosis have a better chance of pregnancy than those with chronic inflammation or endometriosis, which are more frequently associated with secondary infertility (Donnez & Casanas-Roux, 1986).

Obliterative Fibrosis

In obliterative fibrosis, collagen fibres are deposited medial to the inner longitudinal layer of the myosalpinx, resulting in complete occlusion of the lumen. There is minimal involvement of the tubal muscle so there are no palpable or visible nodules. Fortier and Haney (1985) believe that obliterative fibrosis is the commonest cause of proximal occlusion and that it represents a non-specific reaction to injury or inflammation in the interstitial or isthmic segments of the tube.

Fig. 2.3.1a shows a completely closed lumen due to replacement of the epithelium by fibrous connective tissue. The tubal mucosa of the proximal isthmic segment adjacent to the block may be normal (Fig. 2.3.1b), or there may be formation of fibrous polypi (Fig. 2.3.1c).

Chronic Tubal Inflammation

There is evidence of chronic inflammation in up to 40% of obstructed intramural or isthmic segments. The inflammatory process may involve all three layers, causing the epithelium to become atrophic, the submucosal layer dense, and the myosalpinx thickened. The inflammatory lesions are confined to the proximal tube in mild infection, but in severe infections there may also be distal involvement producing fimbrial adhesions, agglutination of the ampullary folds or hydrosalpinx.

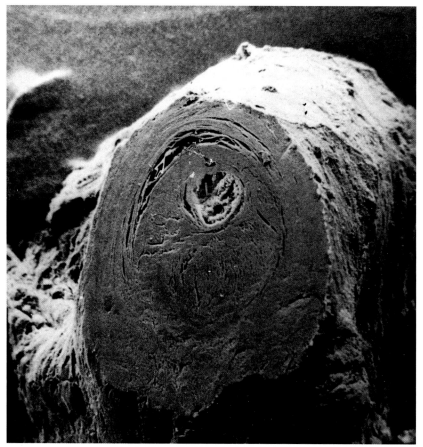

Fig. 2.3.1a–c Isthmic blockage.
a SEM of a transverse section showing marked thickening of the circular muscle layer and adhesions partially occluding the lumen (×20).

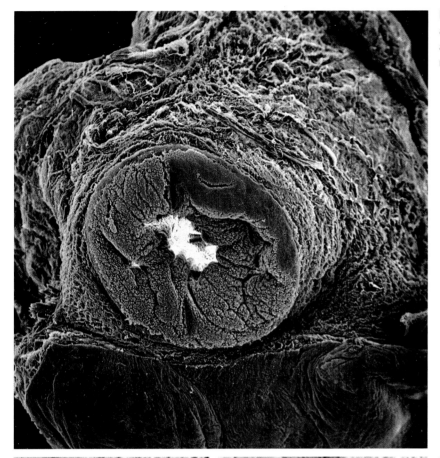

b SEM of a transverse section of isthmus adjacent to the isthmic blockage, showing an apparently normal muscle layer, and mucus in the tubal lumen (×50).

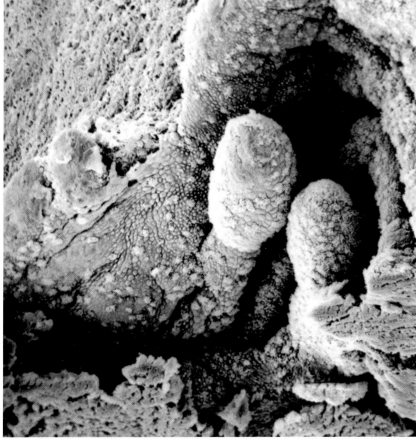

c SEM of a section of the cornu adjacent to the isthmus, showing two intraluminal polyps directed cranially towards the isthmus (×200).

Salpingitis Isthmica Nodosa

The incidence of salpingitis isthmica nodosa varies according to race, from 0.5% in Caucasians to 11% in Jamaican negroes. It is found most frequently in women who have previously had an ectopic pregnancy, and in up to 70% of those undergoing tubal surgery for proximal obstruction (Salat-Baroux *et al.*, 1980).

In salpingitis isthmica nodosa, the wall of the isthmus is thickened with one or more, white or yellow/brown nodules up to 2 cm in diameter (Fig. 2.3.2) which in cross-section have a honeycomb appearance (Figs 2.3.3a & 2.3.3b). Histological examination of the isthmic wall reveals glandular formations. These are lined with epithelium similar to that of the normal tubal mucosa and are surrounded by hyperplastic and hypertrophied muscle fibres (Fig. 2.3.3c). Although some authors (Dougherty, 1968) claim that the glandular islands in the tubal muscle are separate from the underlying mucosa, others (Haines & Taylor, 1975) have demonstrated that many of them do connect with the tubal lumen and are genuine diverticula. Radiological studies have shown branching channels radiating from the main lumen into the myosalpinx, which confirms this theory (Persaud, 1970).

Salpingitis isthmica nodosa has been thought to be the sequel of gonorrhoea, tuberculosis or non-specific infection, but not all patients show evidence of an

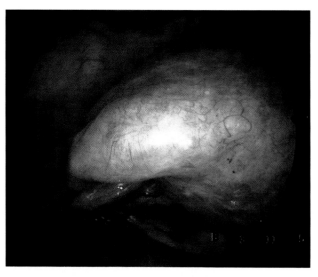

Fig. 2.3.2 **Salpingitis isthmica nodosa resulting in a thickening of the tubal wall.**

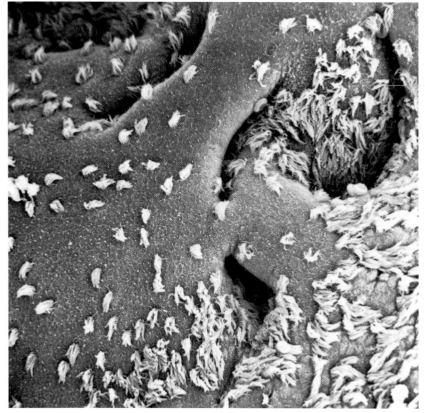

Fig. 2.3.3a–c **Salpingitis isthmica nodosa.**
a SEM showing the tubal mucosa at the isthmo-ampullary junction with intraluminal bridges and formation of pseudoglandular spaces. Note the scarcity of ciliated cells on the bridges and the flat cells with indistinct borders in non-ciliated areas (×500).

inflammatory reaction in the fallopian tube. Park (1978) suggests that it could result from a congenital or developmental defect causing the mesodermal cells in the wall of the tube to differentiate into epithelial cells, whereas Honore and O'Hara (1978) consider that salpingitis isthmica nodosa may be an acquired form of diverticulosis caused by chronic spasm of the isthmic muscle.

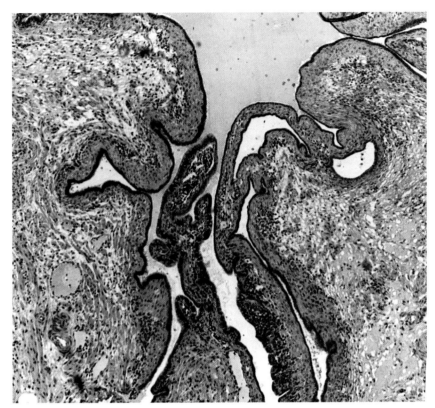

b Light optical microscopic (LOM) section through the isthmus showing the invaginations of the principal lumen lined by extensions of tubal epithelium (×80).

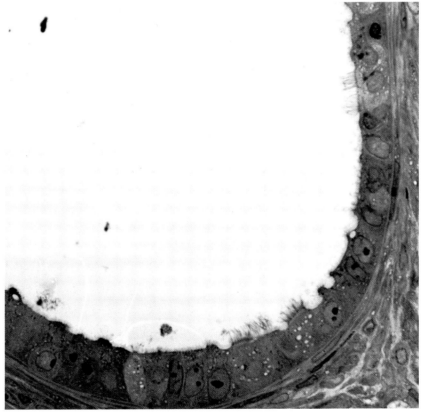

c LOM section through the isthmus showing cuboidal epithelium lining the invagination. Note the marked basal bodies and cytoplasmic vacuoles of the ciliated cells, and the rounded nuclei, conspicuous nucleoli and flat surfaces of the non-ciliated cells (×800).

Endometriosis

Endometriosis of the patent fallopian tube is uncommon, but in proximal tubal obstruction, islands of endometrium replacing the normal mucosa may be found in up to 19% of patients (Fortier & Haney, 1985). The endometrium penetrates the myosalpinx producing an appearance similar to endosalpingeal diverticulosis and, indeed, this may be a manifestation of salpingitis isthmica nodosa.

Tubocornual Polyps

Tubocornual polyps are evident in 2–6% of hysterosalpingograms of infertile patients (Corette, 1977), but their incidence is probably higher as they have been recorded in 11% of hysterectomy and autopsy studies (Lisa *et al.*, 1954). These polyps usually occur in the intramural portion of the tube and are rare in the isthmus (Fig. 2.3.4). They may arise from the endometrium or tubal mucosa, or they may have a fibrous origin. Their association with infertility is, however, debatable.

Polyps at the tubal meatus can be removed hysteroscopically using laser or coagulating forceps, but those occurring in the intramural portion of the tube or isthmus require microsurgical removal or prolonged therapy with danazol.

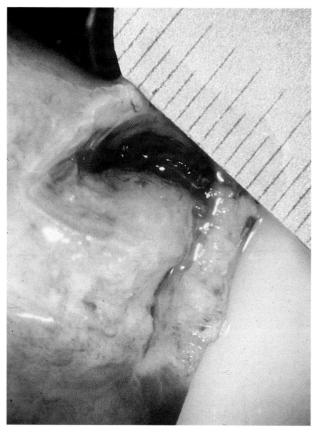

Fig. 2.3.4a–c Large intramural polyp.
a The polyp shown at microsurgery.

b SEM showing the polyp projecting from the mucosa of the intramural lumen (×20).

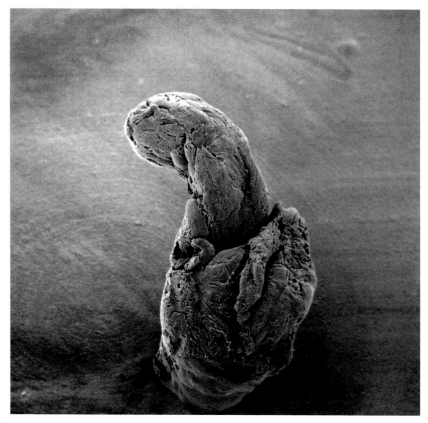

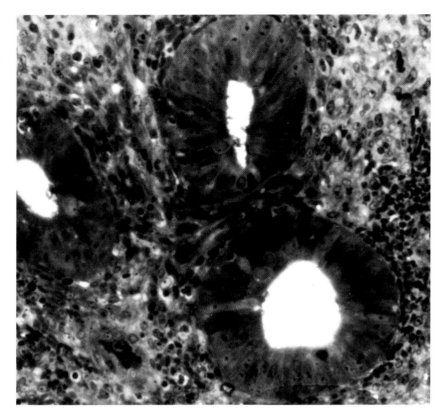

c LOM section through the polyp showing endometrial glands and stroma (×500).

2.4 TUBERCULOSIS

Incidence

The incidence of genital tuberculosis varies with both the population studied and their geographical location but, in general, it has become less common in recent years. In the last 30 years this decrease has been a consequence of the lower incidence of pulmonary and other forms of the disease. In France, between 1961 and 1978, Boury-Heyler (1979) found genital tuberculosis in 5–10% of women with tubal infertility, whereas in a more recent study in the United States, Siegler (1984) found that less than 1% of infertile patients had tuberculosis. Nevertheless, in developing countries tuberculosis remains an important aetiological factor and is found in up to 20% of infertile women.

Pathogenesis

Genital tuberculosis occurs almost always secondary to a focus in another organ, usually the lung, from which it spreads via the bloodstream. Tuberculosis may also spread to the genital tract via the lymphatic circulation, or directly from the peritoneal cavity, urinary tract or bowel, while infection in the genital tract may spread to the peritoneum.

The fallopian tubes are the commonest site of initial infection in genital tuberculosis and it is probable that infection of the endometrium, myometrium, cervix and vagina is due to spread from a focus in the tubes. The disease rarely produces significant symptoms in the early stages and is usually detected during the investigation of infertility, the first signs being demonstrated by hysterosalpingography. It has been estimated that 60–98% of patients with genital tuberculosis are infertile (Woodruff & Pauerstein, 1969).

Gross Pathology

Tuberculosis occurs most often in the ampulla of the tube. Infection of the intramural and isthmic segments is uncommon. At laparotomy, the tube feels rigid on palpation and the ampulla may be dilated, but the fimbriae usually appear normal and the ostium is open. If adhesions develop between the tube and ovary they either close the fimbrial end and cause complete distal occlusion, or cause constriction of the proximal end of the dilated ampulla, resulting in a characteristic 'tobacco pouch' appearance at hysterosalpingography. The general appearance is similar to that of non-tuberculous chronic salpingitis, except in those rare cases which are secondary to peritoneal tuberculosis when there are foci on the serosal surface. The infection is usually limited to the mucosa, but caseating granulomata may extend into the tubal wall, resulting in focal calcification. In tuberculous pyosalpinx, there is a necrotic, cheesy exudate in the lumen of the tube.

Microscopy and Scanning Electron Microscopy

The histological diagnosis is clear when typical tubercles with giant cells and/or caseation are seen in the mucosal folds, and acid-alcohol fast bacilli are demonstrated on Ziehl–Nielsen staining. Occasionally these features, including the demonstration of acid and alcohol fast bacilli, may be absent and the histological picture is similar to that of non-tuberculous chronic salpingitis. An adenomatous pattern in the mucosal folds is highly suggestive of tuberculosis, although it is often associated with other forms of 'irritation' of the mucosa. The appearance of the mucosal folds varies; they may be completely absent or atrophic, or they

may be agglutinated and adhesions may be present. There is also a wide variation in the degree of desquamation and cilial damage (Fig. 2.4.1a, b & c).

De Brux (1971) found that tubercular lesions in the tubes were seldom uniform and were bilateral in 44% of cases. The mucosa was always involved, but 25% of cases also showed evidence of infection in the myosalpinx, and 31% of infection in the serosa. Follicular tuberculosis is the most common form of the disease, followed by fibrocaseous and caseous forms. The exudative form occurs in less than 10% of cases.

Prognosis

The healing process results either in a totally obliterated tubal lumen with infertility, or in scarring of the endosalpinx with markedly decreased fertility. Indeed, term pregnancies following medical or conservative surgical treatment are extremely uncommon, and if pregnancy does occur there is a high risk of tubal implantation.

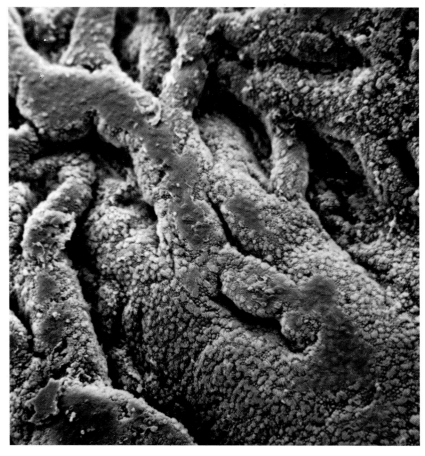

Fig. 2.4.1a–c Tuberculosis of the ampullary mucosa.

a SEM showing that the resulting thick-walled hydrosalpinx has an adenomatous fold pattern forming pseudoglandular spaces. Note the thick covering of exudate in some areas (× 130).

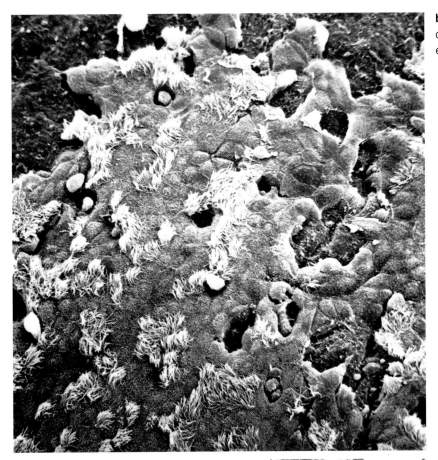

b SEM showing desquamation and deciliation of cells together with loss of epithelium (×500).

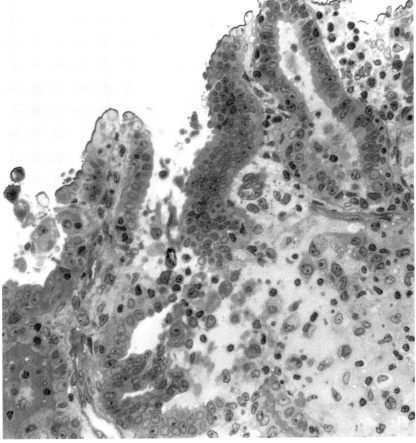

c Post-scanning section showing columnar and pseudostratified epithelia forming inclusions and pseudoglandular spaces, with a marked chronic inflammatory cell infiltrate (LOM, ×500).

2.5 TUBAL PREGNANCY

Incidence

Ectopic pregnancy occurs as often as 1 in 300 live births and the incidence appears to be increasing. Approximately one third of patients are nulliparous and subsequently more than 50% of them will be infertile. An increased awareness of the condition by both patients and doctors, together with the use of new diagnostic methods, means that the diagnosis can often be made before the tube has ruptured, and conservative tubal surgery can be performed. The increasing frequency of diagnosis of tubal pregnancy before rupture in the last 20 years is shown in Fig. 2.5.1 (Brosens *et al.*, 1984).

Pathogenesis

There is considerable variation in the literature regarding the aetiology of ectopic pregnancy. Many causes have been suggested including congenital anomalies of the tube, adhesions, surgical trauma, transmigration of the ovum, tubal spasm, endometriosis and delayed ovulation. A number of risk factors which will delay or arrest the passage of the fertilized ovum both in the tube and in the trophoblast can be defined.

Congenital Defects
De Brux and Dupre-Froment (1961) found acquired or congenital structural abnormalities in 70% of their cases. Congenital defects include hypoplasia of the tube, localized narrowing of the lumen, diverticula, accessory lumina and ostia, and abnormally long tubes. In some cases, there may be evidence of the sequelae of infection in addition to a congenital defect.

Infection
Chronic pelvic infection is generally thought to be the most common underlying cause of the histologically-proven salpingitis found in 30–50% of women with ectopic pregnancies (Niles & Clark, 1969). The causative organisms include *Neisseria gonorrhoeae* and *Mycobacterium tuberculosis*, but it is now being recognized that *Chlamydia trachomatis* is responsible for an increasing proportion of cases. Non-specific infection with other organisms such as *Escherichia coli* is common.

Mild pelvic inflammatory disease seems to be a condition confined to humans and this may be why other mammals seldom develop ectopic pregnancies, despite the capability of their ova to implant outside the uterus under laboratory conditions. The increasing incidence of sexually transmitted disease, with resulting tubal epithelial damage, may be a cause of the increasing incidence of ectopic gestation.

On the other hand, Woodruff and Pauerstein (1969) found that salpingitis isthmica nodosa and follicular salpingitis were responsible for approximately 33% of their cases of tubal pregnancy. They also described changes in the serosa associated with chronic salpingitis, such as the presence of nidi of squamous metaplasia (Walthard's islets) in the peritoneum.

Deciliation
Using scanning electron microscopy Vasquez *et al.* (1983), described deciliation in patients with ectopic pregnancy or a history of ectopic pregnancy. Loss of ciliated cells from the ampulla probably delays the passage of the ovum towards the uterine cavity, resulting in tubal implantation of the embryo after the trophoblast has formed. This could explain why the commonest site of ectopic pregnancy is in the mid-ampulla, and why implantation is less common in the isthmus, and rare in the fimbriae and cornua.

Deciliation is the most characteristic feature of the epithelial cells of the fimbriae and the ampulla in ectopic

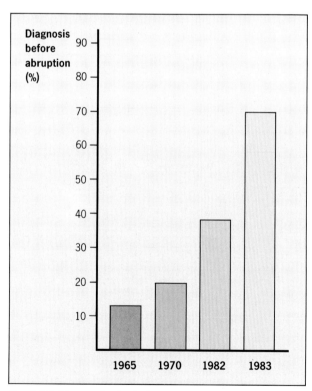

Fig. 2.5.1 Diagnosis of tubal pregnancy.
The frequency with which tubal pregnancy is diagnosed prior to tubal abruption has increased from 12% to 70% between 1965 and 1983. (From Brosens, 1984).

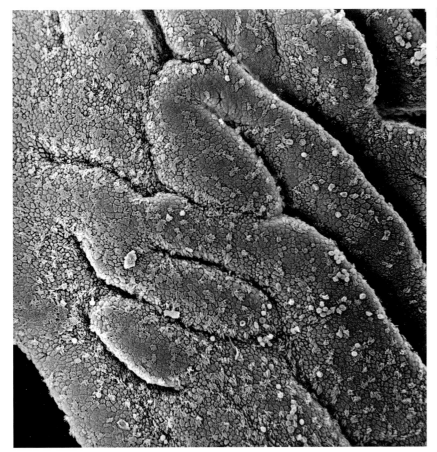

Fig. 2.5.2a–c Ampullary tubal pregnancy at 6 weeks.
a SEM showing paucity of ciliated cells on the mucosal surface (× 250).

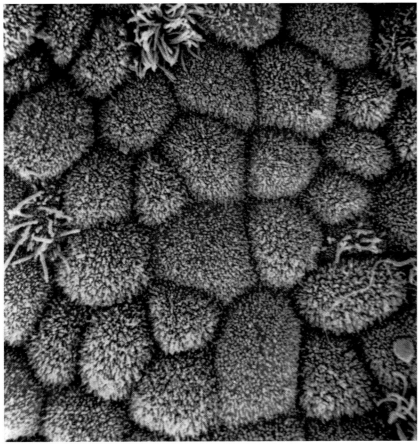

b SEM showing the mucosal surface with densely packed microvilli on the non-ciliated cells. Note also two normally ciliated cells and three with abnormally short cilia (× 1800).

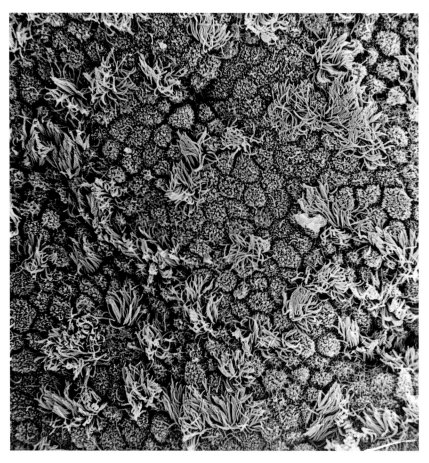

Fig. 2.5.2 continued.
c SEM showing the mucosal surface with ciliated cells representing 20% of the surface area (×1000).

pregnancy, and is more pronounced when the embryo is implanted in these sites than when nidation is in the isthmus (Fig. 2.5.2 a, b & c). This could suggest that the embryo implants at the site of maximal damage or, alternatively, that the hormones produced by the conceptus may have a local influence on deciliation.

Brosens and Vasquez (1976) have found loss of cilia following salpingitis and also in hydrosalpinx, which is generally considered to be a sequel of infection. Sloughing of the ciliated cells occurs during the acute stage of salpingitis and their permanent loss can only be avoided by prompt, appropriate antibiotic therapy. Although chronic inflammation has only been reported in approximately 40% of oviducts with an ectopic pregnancy, the deciliation in the apparently normal fallopian tubes may well be the result of a previous inflammatory process. The fact that the contralateral tube also shows deciliation is more in keeping with an inflammatory process affecting both oviducts, as is the high recurrence rate of tubal pregnancy in the contralateral tube after salpingectomy for a first tubal pregnancy. The recurrence rate is higher in patients with a previous history of pelvic inflammatory disease, septic abortion or postpartum endometritis.

In ectopic pregnancy, the mucosal folds are still present at the site of implantation, but are more widely separated and flattened. In the flattened folds, the altered cells are both numerous and distended, and appear to squeeze the cilia of the neighbouring cells. Common characteristic findings in the tubal mucosa of ectopic pregnancy include polyhedral cells and desquamated cells, and cells bearing few, or drooping cilia (Fig. 2.5.3a, b & c). Using light microscopy, Birch and Collins (1961) observed squamous transformation similar to that found in the endometrium at the site of intrauterine implantation. They also noted the presence of cellular hyperplasia, producing polyp-like formations in the tube containing the ectopic pregnancy, and sprouts of proliferating trophoblast can be seen protruding on the surface mucosa of the implantation area (Fig. 2.5.4a, b & c)

Mitotic figures in the epithelium, an extremely rare finding in a normal fallopian tube, have been found in some tubes containing a tubal pregnancy and are probably related to attempted repair or regeneration.

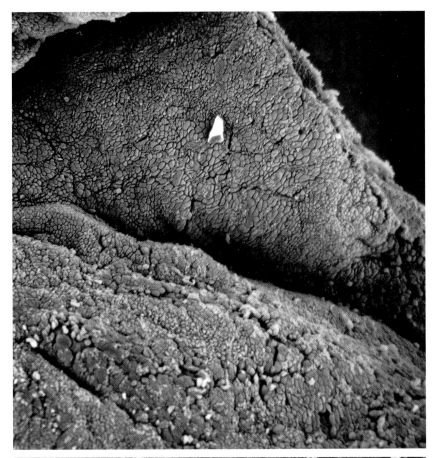

Fig. 2.5.3a–c Recurrent tubal pregnancy.
a SEM of the fimbriae shows extensive deciliation (×200).

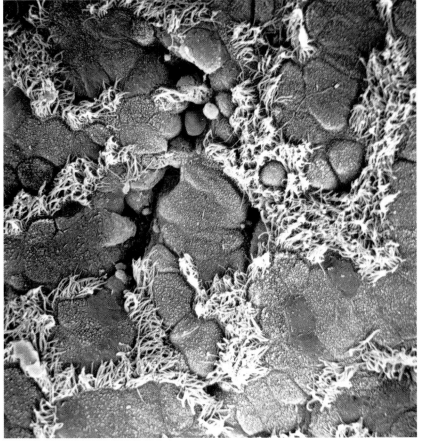

b SEM showing the fimbrial cells with irregular outlines and 73% surface deciliation (×1000).

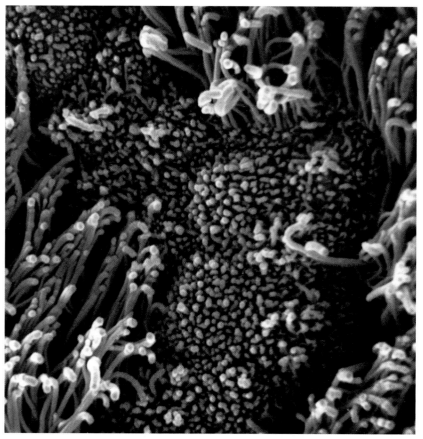

Fig. 2.5.3 continued.
c SEM showing clubbing of the cilial tips, and the rounded and elongated villi of the non-ciliated cells (×5200).

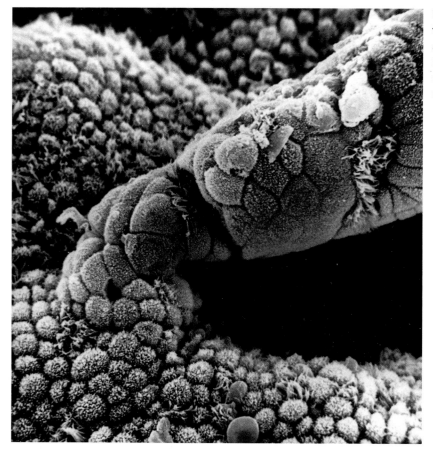

Fig. 2.5.4a–c The ampullary mucosa at the implantation site.
a SEM showing a polypoid formation with large flattened epithelial cells bearing microvilli which have arisen from the mucosal surface (×850).

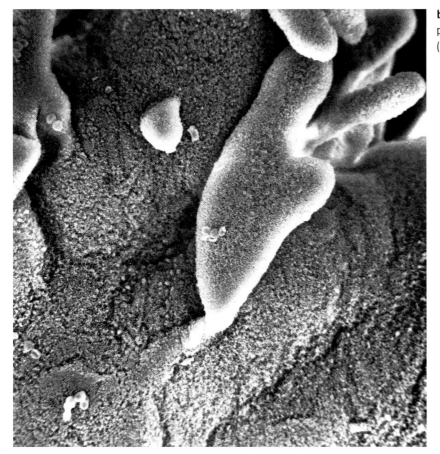

b SEM showing sprouts of trophoblast projecting into the epithelial surface (×280).

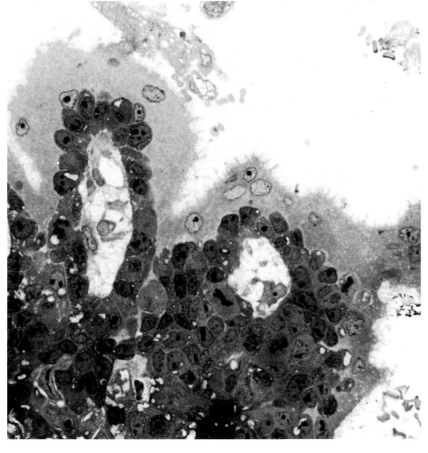

c Post-scanning section through the villi showing syncytiotrophoblast with microvilli, cytotrophoblast with mitosis, and the stromal core. Mitotic figures can be seen in the cytotrophoblast (LOM, ×1000).

Endometrialization

Endometrialization and decidual transformation of the mucosa have been reported in association with tubal pregnancy and are possible aetiological factors on the basis that they increase its receptivity to the fertilized ovum. However, Novak and Woodruff (1967) do not consider that these features are important because, firstly, portions of tubal mucosa resembling endometrium have been described in normal fertile women and, secondly, the decidual reaction has been found in the tubal mucosa of normal intrauterine pregnancies. Furthermore, decidualization of the mucosa tends to inhibit nidation (Noyes, 1959), and decidual changes normally occur only after implantation.

Decidualization of the stromal cells underlying the epithelium may be found in tubal pregnancy, but is poorly developed compared to the stromal response in the endometrium of an intrauterine pregnancy. Woodruff and Pauerstein (1969) described decidualization at the implantation site in one third of their cases of ectopic pregnancy, and found no increase in the number of muscle fibres although hypertrophy of the tubal muscularis has been described.

Surgical Trauma

A history of previous tubal surgery and previous ectopic pregnancy are high risk factors for tubal pregnancy. After reviewing the literature relating to the incidence of ectopic pregnancy following failure of different types of tubal sterilization, McCausland (1980) concluded that the risk of tuboperitoneal fistula formation was higher with the more destructive methods, such as electrocoagulation, than with mechanical methods, such as clips and silicone rings, which destroy less tissue and do not open the tubal lumen. These small fistulae permit sperm to enter the peritoneal cavity and find their way to a recently released oöcyte.

Stock and Nelson (1984) postulate that following sterilization the fluid dynamics in the remaining tubal segments determine the site of implantation of a pregnancy. They deny the importance given to endometrialization, the luminal diameter of the proximal tuboperitoneal fistula, the 'recanalization' hypothesis (Honore & O'Hara, 1978) and the 'endosalpingoblastosis' concept (McCausland, 1982).

Contraceptive Techniques

The use of intrauterine contraceptive devices (IUCDs) and the related increased incidence of subclinical pelvic inflammatory disease also increases the risk of tubal pregnancy. Although it has been suggested that these devices inhibit intrauterine implantation, it is unlikely that they have any influence on tubal or ovarian implantation, apart from their association with pelvic inflammatory disease. A tubal inflammatory infiltrate has been reported in 25–47% of women using IUCDs, but recent studies have failed to culture any microorganism from most of these fallopian tubes, which suggests that the inflammatory reaction is due to the contraceptive method (Collins *et al.*, 1984).

Other contraceptive methods associated with an increased risk of ectopic pregnancy are the low-dose progestogen pill and postcoital oestrogens. Treatment with progestogens has been associated with decreased numbers of ciliated cells and this might be the underlying cause for the ectopic gestations in women receiving these drugs.

Abnormal Conceptus

Woodruff and Pauerstein (1969) suggest that some of the causes of extrauterine pregnancy are associated with the conceptus. These include external and internal transmigration of the ovum, delayed ovulation, excessive numbers of abnormal sperm and anomalies of the fertilized ovum, such as chromosomal abnormalities.

Summary of Aetiological Factors

Despite considerable research, the relative importance of the aetiological factors in tubal pregnancy remains controversial, and many authors have found no apparent abnormality in the fallopian tube containing an ectopic pregnancy in a significant number of their cases.

Site

Approximately 60–80% of ectopic pregnancies implant in the ampulla, 15–30% in the isthmus, and 5% in the fimbriae and intramural segments (Fox & Buckley, 1982). Persaud (1970) studied the radiological and histological patterns of the oviducts removed at surgery for tubal pregnancy. He suggested that implantation in the ampulla and fimbriae was caused by the sequelae of infection, and that isthmic and intramural implantations were more often associated with congenital defects.

Evolution

Implantation in the human is always interstitial (Fig. 2.5.5), but placentation in the tube has received little attention in the current literature. Ectopic pregnancy can result in tubal abortion, resorption of the conceptus, so-called rupture of the tube, or advanced abdominal pregnancy. The result may well depend on whether implantation occurs on the mesenteric or the antimesenteric side of the fallopian tube. The major supply arteries are on the mesenteric side, whereas the antimesenteric side is supplied by their small terminal branches. The trophoblast is more likely to survive if it implants on the mesenteric side, as implantation on the antimesenteric side may lead to early death of the conceptus with resorption or tubal abortion.

If the embryo continues to develop there is a remarkable similarity between the trophoblastic migration in the tubal wall and that found in the uterine wall following a normal implantation. In the first few weeks of an intrauterine pregnancy, a wave of intra-arterial trophoblast invades the walls of the decidual spiral arteries and migrates retrogradely along them. This invasion is associated with loss of musculoelastic tissue and its replacement by fibrinoid material and intramural trophoblast (Pijnenborg *et al.*, 1981). In the uterus, the arteries are able to distend without rupture because they are supported by the surrounding decidualized tissue or myometrium. In the fallopian tube however, they are more likely to rupture when the distension extends to involve the arteries outside the myosalpinx where they are supported only by loose connective tissue. Bleeding from these small arteries and consequent haematoma formation, rather than rupture of the tube by the expanding conceptus, may be the major cause of so-called 'tubal rupture' which usually occurs at 8–10 weeks' gestation.

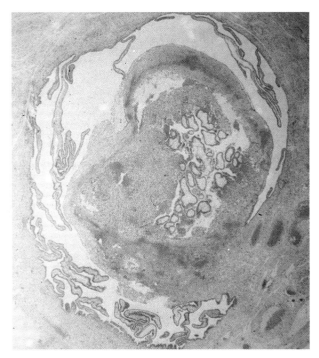

Fig. 2.5.5 Tubal pregnancy.
Section at the site of implantation showing the pregnancy implanted in the tubal wall and the lumen distorted by the pregnancy. (Courtesy of Dr H. Evers.)

2.6 POSTSTERILIZATION

Tubal sterilization has been used as a method of permanent contraception for more than 100 years and has been gaining world-wide popularity for the last 20 years. There are more than 100 different methods but those commonly used in the last decade include tubal ligation, laparoscopic electrocoagulation and, more recently, application of silicone rings and tubal clips.

The increasing number of sterilizations being performed on relatively young women of low parity, together with the more widespread availability of tubal microsurgery, has led to a greatly increased demand for reversal during the past 10 years. There is therefore a renewed interest in the changes which occur in the fallopian tubes following sterilization.

Radiological Studies

Radiological studies of women who have been sterilized have demonstrated changes in the fallopian tube away from the site of occlusion. Examples of such changes include blockage of the tubal ostium, diverticula and dilatation of the intramural portion. These have not

been found in control women of similar age (Querleu *et al.*, 1983). Polyps and fistulae also occur with a prevalence which increases with time; post-sterilization studies have demonstrated abnormalities in 28% of tubes after 3 years, rising to 72% after 10 years (Vasquez *et al.*, 1980).

Histopathology

Histological changes have been found in the tubal segments remaining after sterilization. These include flattening and fibrosis of the mucosal folds, deciliation, polyp formation, tuboperitoneal fistulae and tubal endometriosis.

Deciliation
In the blind loop of tube resulting from ligation the mucosal folds may be absent and there may also be generalized deciliation (Fig. 2.6.1). The deciliation is probably progressive and depends on the degree of dilatation of the obstructed tubal segment. Bernhardt-Huth *et al.* (1981), suggested that deciliation and other

mucosal changes could be related to local damage to the tubal blood supply resulting from the sterilization procedure. This could lead to an insufficient local level of ovarian steroid hormones for the maintenance of the normal tubal mucosa. However data pertaining to the serum levels of ovarian steroids following sterilization are conflicting and no studies have been performed on their local levels. If deciliation is due to hormone deficiency, it should be more generalized and would affect the distal tube close to the site of the occlusion rather than be confined to the proximal segment where, in any case, the deciliation is patchy.

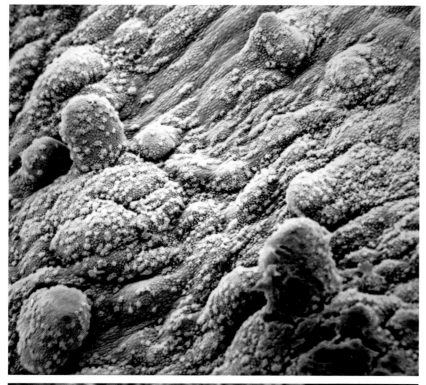

Fig. 2.6.1a & b Isthmic segment of the uterine side of a fallopian tubal block 5 years after Pomeroy tubal ligation.
a SEM showing flattened mucosa, areas of deciliation and three polyps (×125).

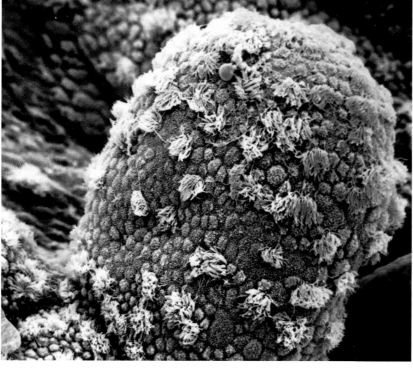

b SEM showing that the surface of the polyp with ciliated and non-ciliated cells is in continuity with the luminal epithelium (×630).

Polyps
The polyps are usually small but can be easily seen with the operating microscope. Their epithelium and stroma are similar to that in the surrounding tube (Fig. 2.6.2a), but occasionally the epithelium may be glandular suggesting that some of the polyps are derived from foci of acquired endometriosis (Fig. 2.6.2b). The cause of polyp formation is not fully understood, but current theories include the ability of the tubal mucosa to proliferate, and the possibility of an inflammatory reaction in the stroma following the accumulation of retrograde menstrual debris.

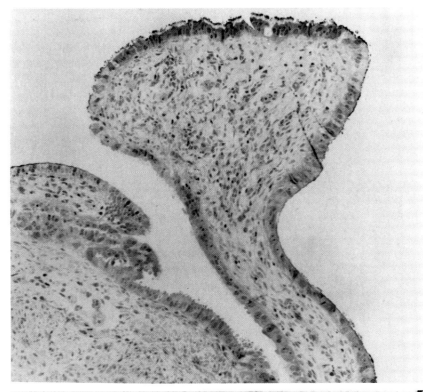

Fig. 2.6.2a & b Isthmic polyp.
a LOM showing that the epithelium and stroma of the polyp are similar to that in the surrounding tube (×200).

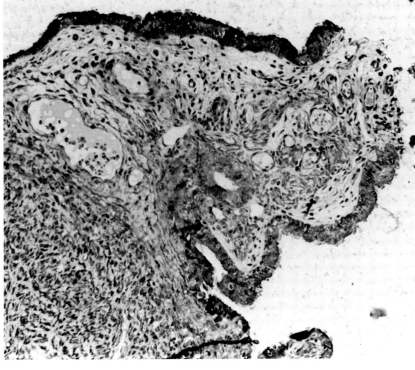

b LOM showing glandular structures suggestive of an endometrial origin (×200).

Fistulae

Tubo-peritoneal fistulae are most common in women who have been sterilized by electrocautery when the length of the proximal segment is less than 4 cm and the postoperative interval is more than 3 years (Rock *et al.*, 1981). Tubo-peritoneal fistulae also occur after ligature of the ampulla and after fimbriectomy, and are probably due to the traumatic effect of the ligature on the tubal wall which has been weakened by the formation of a hydrosalpinx (Metz, 1979).

Tubal Endometriosis

Several investigators have found endometriosis in the fallopian tube following sterilization, particularly after electrocautery and also after application of silastic

rings (Stock, 1982; Donnez *et al.*, 1984). Other investigators have, however, failed to confirm these findings (Robinson & Filshie, 1984).

Clinical Significance

There is no correlation between the success of micro-surgical reversal and the time elapsed since sterilization. There is, however, a correlation between tubal lesions and subsequent fertility. In one study, 50% of the women who achieved term pregnancy following reversal, had normal proximal tubal segments on one or both sides (Vasquez *et al.*, 1980), whereas all of the women who failed to become pregnant had abnormal proximal segments.

2.7   CONGENITAL TUBAL ANOMALIES

Congenital abnormalities or anatomical distortion of otherwise patent tubes are not common and their clinical significance is not always clear.

Convoluted or Tortuous Tubes

Convoluted but patent fallopian tubes can be diagnosed by hysterosalpingography or laparoscopy. This abnormality was studied by Moore-White (1960) who obtained histological evidence of aplasia of the myosalpinx. The tubal abnormality is frequently associated with elongation of the fimbria ovarica, which may be more than 4 cm in length, and also with polycystic ovarian disease. The elongation of the fimbria ovarica may be due to the pulling and stretching of the supporting muscular ligaments by the large, heavy gonads.

Salpingoscopy shows dilatation of the thin-walled tubal lumen with distended and flattened mucosal folds, similar to those seen in thin-walled hydrosalpinx (Fig. 2.7.1). Progression of the salpingoscope in a convoluted tube can be difficult because of the acute bends in the lumen. Convoluted tubes are compatible with fertility.

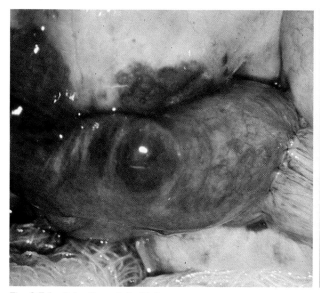
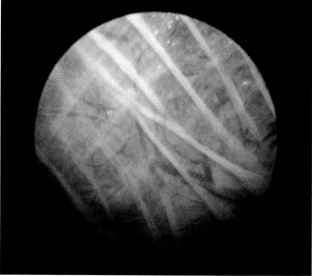

Fig. 2.7.1a & b   Convoluted tube.
a Localized thin-walled distension seen at laparotomy.

b Salpingoscopy shows a transparent tubal wall with poor vascularization and widely separated mucosal folds.

Accessory Tubes and Accessory Ostia

Accessory tubes are small, non-patent cylindrical structures attached to the ampulla of a normal sized tube. At their distal end there is a small fimbria-like structure lined with ciliated epithelium. The high incidence of these structures suggests that they are too common to be considered pathological. They may however contribute to infertility (Beyth & Kopolovic, 1982) as the ova may be captured by the fimbriae of the accessory, occluded fallopian tube instead of the main one and, if fertilization occurs here, an ectopic pregnancy will result. Therefore, whenever these structures are encounterd during pelvic surgery, particularly in infertile women, they should be removed.

Accessory ostia are always located on the anti-mesenteric border of the ampullary segment of the fallopian tube but their incidence is not known. Cohen (1987) has recommended their closure by microsurgery to restore both the normal ovum conduction mechanism and the environment for fertilization and cleavage (Fig. 2.7.2).

Segmental Obstruction

Segmental obstruction is a rare finding which has been seen in the middle third of the ampulla on two occasions in our experience. In both cases there was an ectopic pregnancy in the contralateral tube (Fig. 2.7.3).

The Immotile Cilia Syndrome

The Immotile Cilia Syndrome (ICS) is characterized by congenitally non-functioning cilia and is analogous to a condition which occurs in men with a long history of chronic and recurrent infections in the upper and lower respiratory tract. These men have a reduced tracheo-bronchial clearance which probably leads to stasis of secretions and a resultant predisposition to infection, and produce living spermatozoa with straight immotile tails which render them either non-motile or capable of only feeble movements (Afzelius *et al.*, 1975).

Afzelius *et al.* (1978), have reported on six women with ICS; they found no history of ectopic pregnancy

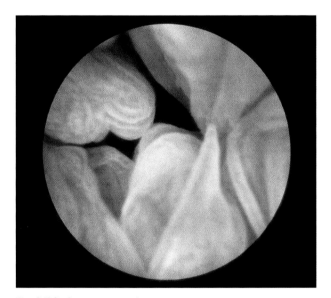

Fig. 2.7.2 Accessory ostium.
Salpingoscopic view of the mucosa.

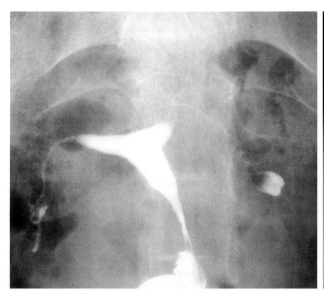

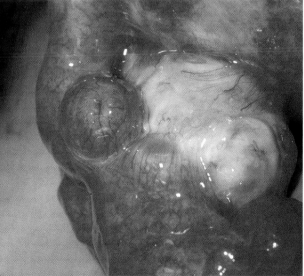

Fig. 2.7.3a & b Segmental obstruction.
a Radiological view of segmental obstruction of the left tube.
Right salpingectomy was performed for ruptured tubal pregnancy.

b View of the obstructed segment at tubal reconstructive surgery.

or salpingitis, and two of the women had had children. Rott (1979) found evidence in the literature to suggest that such women have reduced fertility, presumably due to lack of cilial activity in the tubal mucosa.

ICS is inherited in an autosomal manner, the primary gene product being either a dynein or another component residing in dynein arms, a protein which binds dynein to the microtubular tubulines, or a defect in the transport of dynein from the site of synthesis to the site of action. This is consistent with the fact that some patients with ICS have dynein arms but have defects in the central tubule-sheet complex, which suggests the possibility of different gene products.

ICS includes, but is not identical with, Kartagener's syndrome, in which there is situs inversus, bronchiectasis and chronic sinusitis; thus some patients with

ICS also have the Kartagener triad. It can therefore be assumed that ICS is not a single entity, but that many gradations may exist between a fully functioning ciliary system and a completely non-functioning system, and this may be related to the ultrastructural basis of the disease.

Indeed, it has been demonstrated that not all patients have immotile cilia, but that the ciliary beat is abnormal due to 'primary cilial dyskinesia' resulting in a more difficult diagnosis of the syndrome. Furthermore, architectural defects of bronchial cilia such as megacilia, disorganized cilia and disorganized axonemes have been reported in children with recurrent pulmonary infections, the anomalies regressing after prolonged antibiotic therapy, suggesting an acquired origin (Corbeel *et al.*, 1981).

REFERENCES

Afzelius, B.A., Eliasson, R., Johnsen, O. & Lindholmer, C. (1975) Lack of dynein arms in immotile human spermatozoa. *Journal of Cell Biology*, **66**, 225–232.

Afzelius, B.A., Camner, P. & Mossberg, B. (1978) On the function of cilia in the female reproductive tract. *Fertility and Sterility*, **29**, 72–74.

Bernhardt-Huth, D., Frantzen, C.H. & Schlosser, H.W. (1981) Morphology of rabbit oviduct after microsurgical techniques for reanastomosis of the isthmus or ampulla. *Archives of Gynecology*, **230**, 251–262.

Beyth, Y. & Kopolovic, J. (1982) Accessory tubes: a possible contributory factor in fertility. *Fertility and Sterility*, **38**, 382–383.

Birch, H.W. & Collins, C.G. (1961) Atypical changes of genital epithelium associated with ectopic pregnancy. *Americal Journal of Obstetrics and Gynecology*, **81**, 1198–1208.

Boury-Heyler, C. (1979) La tuberculose tubaire, aspect actuel en France. In: *Oviduct et Fertilite*. Edited by I. Brosens, M. Cognat, A. Constantin & M. Thibier. pp.219–230. Paris: Masson.

Brosens, I.A. & Vasquez, G. (1976) Fimbrial microbiopsy. *Journal of Reproductive Medicine*, **16**, 171–178.

Brosens, I., Gordts, S., Vasquez, G. & Boeckx, W. (1985) Function-retaining surgical management of ectopic pregnancy. *European Journal of Obstetrics, Gynecology and Reproductive Biology*, **18**, 395.

Brosens, I., Gordts, S., Vasquez, G. & Boeckx, W. (1985) Function-retaining surgical management of ectopic pregnancy. *European Journal of Obstetrics and Gynecology and Reproductive Biology*, **18**, 395–402.

Cohen, B.M. (1987) Microsurgical reconstruction of congenital tubal anomalies. *Microsurgery*, **8**, 68–77.

Collins, J.A., Gillett, P.G., Perlin, I.A., Embil, J.A., Zayid, I., Richards, G. & Kirk, M.E. (1984) Microbiological and histological findings in the fallopian tubes of women using various contraceptive methods. *Contraception*, **30**, 457–466.

Corbeel, L., Cornillie, F., Lauwerijns, J., Boel, M. & Van Denberghe, G. (1981) Ultrastructural abnormalities of bronchial cilia in children with recurrent airway infections and bronchiectasis. *Archives of Disease in Childhood*, **56**, 929–933.

Corette, L. (1977) La polypose de la portion intramurale de la trompe. Memoire pour l'agregation, Lille.

De Brux, J. & Dupre-Froment, J. (1961) Les anomalies congenitales dans l'histogenese des grossesses extra-uterines. In: *La Grossesse Extra-uterine.* p.89. Paris: Masson.

De Brux, J. (1971) *Histopathologie Gynecologique.* pp.271–298. Paris: Masson.

De Brux, J. (1971) *Histopathologie Gynecologique.* pp.379–393. Paris: Masson.

Donnez, J., Casanas-Roux, F., Ferin, J. & Thomas, K. (1984) Tubal polyps, epithelial inclusions and endometriosis after tubal sterilization. *Fertility and Sterility*, **41**, 564–568.

Donnez, J. & Casanas-Roux, F. (1986) Prognostic factors influencing the pregnancy rate after microsurgical anastomosis. *Fertility and Sterility*, **46**, 1084–1092.

Dougherty, C.M. (1968) *Surgical Pathology of Gynecologic Disease.* pp.425–492. London: Harper & Row.

Drapier, E., Bremond, A. & Rochet, Y. (1979) Les dystophies tubaires et leurs consequences sur la fertilite. In: *Oviducte et Fertilite.* Edited by I. Brosens, M. Cognat, A. Constantin & M. Thibier, pp.205–217. Paris: Masson.

Fortier, K.J. & Haney, A.F. (1985) The pathologic spectrum of uterotubal junction obstruction. *Obstetrics and Gynecology*, **65**, 93–98.

Fox, H. & Buckley, C. (1982) *Pathology for Gynaecologists.* pp.240–245. London: Edward Arnold Publishers Ltd.

Haines, M. & Taylor, C.W. (1975) *Gynaecological Pathology*, 2nd edition. p.397. Edinburgh: Churchill Livingstone.

Honore, L.H. & O'Hara, K.E. (1978) Failed tubal sterilization as an etiologic factor in ectopic tubal pregnancy. *Fertility and Sterility*, **29**, 509–511.

Jacobson, L. & Westrom, L. (1969) Objectivized diagnosis of acute pelvic inflammatory disease. Diagnostic and prognostic value of routine laparoscopy. *American Journal of Obstetrics and Gynecology*, **105**, 1088–1098.

Laufer, N., Simon, A., Schenker, J.G., Sekeles, E. & Cohen, R. (1984) Fallopian tubal mucosal damage induced experimentally by *Escherichia coli* in the rabbit. A scanning electron microscopic study. *Pathology, Research and Practice*, **178**, 605–610.

Lisa, J.R., Gioia, J.D. & Rubin, I.C. (1954) Observations on the interstitial portion of the fallopian tube. *Surgery, Gynecology and Obstetrics*, **99**, 159–169.

McCausland, A. (1980) High rate of ectopic pregnancy following laparoscopic tubal coagulation failures. *American Journal of Obstetrics and Gynecology*, **136**, 97–101.

McCausland, A. (1982) Endosalpingosis ('endosalpingoblastosis') following laparoscopic tubal coagulation as an etiologic factor of ectopic pregnancy. *American Journal of Obstetrics and Gynecology*, **143**, 12–24.

Metz, K.G.P. (1979) Fistules tubo-peritoneales acquises. Frequence, morphologie, causes et consequences sur la fertilite. In: *Oviducte et Fertilite.* Edited by I. Brosens, M. Cognat, A. Constantin & M. Thibier. pp.253–264. Paris: Masson.

Moore-White, M. (1960) Evaluation of tubal plastic operations. *International Journal of Fertility*, **5**, 237–250.

Niles, J.H. & Clark, J.F.H. (1969) Pathogenesis of tubal pregnancy. *American Journal of Obstetrics and Gynecology*, **105**, 1230–1234.

Novak, E.R. & Woodruff, J.D. (1967) *Novak's Gynecologic and Obstetric Pathology*, 6th edition. pp.432–450. Philadelphia: W.B. Saunders Company.

Noyes, R.W. (1959) The underdeveloped secretory endometrium. *American Journal of Obstetrics and Gynecology*, **77**, 929–945.

Park, W.W. (1978) Lesions of the uterine tube. In: *Reversibility of Female Sterilization.* Edited by I. Brosens & R.M.H. Winston. pp.21–30. London: Academic Press.

Persaud, V. (1970) Etiology of ectopic pregnancy. Radiologic and pathologic studies. *Obstetrics and Gynecology*, **36**, 257–263.

Pijnenborg, R., Robertson, W.B., Brosens, I. & Dixon, G. (1981) Trophoblast invasion and the establishment of haemochorial placentation in man and laboratory animals. *Placenta*, **2**, 71–92.

Querleu, D., Bacro, V. & Crepin, C. (1983) Etude radiologique de la portion proximale de la trompe après sterilization. *Gynecologie*, **34**, 27–34.

Robinson, B. & Filshie, G.M. (1984) Histology of human fallopian tube subsequent to sterilization with the Filshie clip: a light and electron microscopy study. Personal communication.

Rock. J.A., Parmley, T.H., King, T.N., Loufe, L.E. & Su, S.C. (1981) Endometriosis and the development of tuboperitoneal fistulas after tubal ligation. *Fertility and Sterility*, **35**, 16.

Rott, H.D. (1979) Kartagener's syndrome and the syndrome of immotile cilia. *Human Genetics*, **46**, 249–261.

Salat-Baroux, J., Cornier, E. & Couturier, J.Y. (1980) Obstruction pathologique de la portion initiale de l'isthme tubaire. Analyse de 50 interventions microchirurgicales. *Journal de Gynecologie, Obstetrique et Biologie de la Reproduction*, **9**, 579–586.

Siegler, A.M. (1984) Female genital tuberculosis and the role of hysterosalpingography. *Infertility*, **7**, 175–186.

Stock, R.J. (1982) Postsalpingectomy endometriosis: a reassessment. *Obstetrics and Gynecology*, **60**, 560–570.

Stock, R.J. & Nelson, K.J. (1984) Ectopic pregnancy subsequent to sterilization: histologic evaluation and clinical implications. *Fertility and Sterility*, **42**, 211–215.

Sweet, R.L., Mills, J., Hadley, K.W., Blumenstock, E., Schachter, J., Robbie, M.O. & Draper, D.L. (1979) Use of laparoscopy to determine the microbiologic etiology of acute salpingitis. *American Journal of Obstetrics and Gynecology*, **134**, 68–74.

Tatum, H.J. & Schmidt, F.H. (1977) Contraceptive and sterilization practices and extrauterine pregnancy: a realistic perspective. *Fertility and Sterility*, **28**, 407–421.

Vasquez, G., Winston, R.M.L., Boeckx, W. & Brosens, I.A. (1980) Tubal lesions subsequent to sterilization and their relation to fertility after attempts at reversal. *American Journal of Obstetrics and Gynecology*, **138**, 86–92.

Vasquez, G., Winston, R.M.L. & Brosens, I.A. (1983) Tubal mucosa in ectopic pregnancy. *British Journal of Obstetrics and Gynaecology*, **90**, 468–474.

Vasquez, G., Vemer, H., Boeckx, W. & Brosens, I.A. (1984) Ciliogenesis following salpingostomy of rabbit hydrosalpinges. *European Journal of Obstetrics and Gynaecoloy and Reproductive Biology*, **18**, 103–118.

Westman, A. (1950) Aetiology, diagnosis and surgical treatment of female sterility. *Acta Obstetrica et Gynecologica Scandinavica*, **30**, 186–202.

Westrom, M.P. (1975) Effect of pelvic inflammatory disease on fertility. *American Journal of Obstetrics and Gynecology*, **121**, 707–713.

Westrom, L., Bengtsson, L.P. & Mardh, P.A. (1976) The risk of pelvic inflammatory disease in women using intrauterine contraceptive devices as compared to non-users. *Lancet*, **2**, 221–224.

Westrom, L. & Mardh, P.A. (1977) Epidemiology, aetiology and prognosis of acute salpingitis in non-gonococcal urethritis and related infections. Edited by D. Hobson & K.K. Holmes. p.84. Washington, DC: American Society of Microbiology.

Westrom, L. (1980) Incidence, prevalence and trends of acute pelvic inflammatory disease, and its consequences in industrialized countries. *American Journal of Obstetrics and Gynaecology*, **138**, 880.

Woodruff, J.D. & Pauerstein, C.J. (1969) *The Fallopian Tube. Structure, Function, Pathology and Management.* Edited by J.D. Woodruff & C.J. Pauerstein. Baltimore: The Williams and Wilkins Co.

3   *ENDOMETRIOSIS*

3.1 THE ROLE OF ENDOMETRIOSIS IN INFERTILITY

Endometriosis is a disease of women, occurring only during the reproductive years. Although its association with infertility is well established, the explanation of its action is one of the most controversial fields in reproductive medicine; thus, the treatment of infertility in many women remains pragmatic.

Endometriosis-Related Infertility

The association between endometriosis and infertility has largely been based on the high incidence of the condition in women undergoing fertility investigation, in whom laparoscopy has revealed its presence in 20–50% of cases. The prevalence of endometriosis in the general population is, however, not known, though estimates of the incidence have been derived from studies made at the time of tubal sterilization (Fig. 3.1.1). These data may not reflect the incidence in infertile women and, moreover, marked differences have been noted between prospective and retrospective studies, suggesting that the variation in incidence may, in part, be influenced by the investigator's level of interest and knowledge of the disease.

Although the cause of infertility is obvious when endometriosis results in extensive tubo-ovarian adhesions or tubal distortion which interfere with ovulation or ovum release and pick-up, there is disagreement on whether endometriosis adversely affects fertility in the absence of mechanical factors. Recent studies from donor insemination programmes support the view that endometriosis is associated with a lower fecundity even when mechanical factors are absent, and the monthly probability of conception in women with endometriosis is 70–80% less than in normal women (Jansen, 1986; Hammond *et al.*, 1986). Similar reduced fecundity rates have been recorded in studies where medical and surgical treatment of infertility have been compared with expectant management, though many of these were retrospective and not corrected for other factors.

More recently, Thomas and Cooke (1987) have been unable to demonstrate that treatment or elimination of mild endometriosis improves future fertility, but have confirmed that although the cumulative pregnancy rate in women with endometriosis is below that of the general population, it is the same as that of women with unexplained infertility. These authors therefore question whether mild endometriosis has a causal role in infertility.

The Possible Causes of Infertility in Endometriosis

When endometriosis is accompanied by normal, patent fallopian tubes and normally functioning ovaries, more subtle and complex explanations must be sought for the associated infertility. These include disturbance of follicular maturation, ovulation, ovum release, ovum pick-up and transport, pre-implantation development, corpus luteum formation, endometrial preparedness, early implantation, peritoneal factors and endometrial autoantibodies.

Indication for Laparoscopy	Incidence of Endometriosis (%)
Interval sterilization	
retrospective	1.4–5
prospective	10–18
Chronic pelvic pain	8.5–47
Unexplained infertility	21–51
Reversal of sterilization	18

Fig. 3.1.1 Incidence of endometriosis at laparoscopy.

Disturbance of Follicular Maturation

Disturbance of follicular maturation in women with endometriosis has been demonstrated by a lower growth rate of follicles (Doody *et al.*, 1988). A low level of luteinizing hormone receptors in the granulosa cells of the Graafian follicle, which fails to increase during the follicular phase of the cycle has also been reported (Kauppila *et al.*,1982; Roennberg *et al.*,1984). However, no significant difference has been found in the fertilizibility of oöcytes from women with endometriosis in *in vitro* fertilization (IVF) programmes. Discrepancies reported in early studies were probably related to prior treatment and different stimulation regimens.

Ovulatory Disturbances

Ovulatory disturbances such as anovulation, luteinization of the unruptured follicle and luteal stage deficiency have been claimed to be factors involved in the infertility associated with endometriosis. Ovulatory defects have been found in 10–27% of such women and Thomas *et al.* (1986) found anovulation in 11% of cases. The incidence of unruptured follicle in women with endometriosis is uncertain and conflicting data may reflect differences in diagnostic techniques. The association between abnormalities of the luteal phase and endometriosis has not been substantiated, and correction of luteal phase defects has not proved successful in the treatment of infertility associated with endometriosis.

The Peritoneal Microenvironment

In recent years the peritoneal microenvironment and its constituents have been studied with renewed interest because of the possibility that prostaglandins, macrophages, immunoglobulins and complement factors in the peritoneal fluid may affect fertility (Schenken & Asch, 1980; Vernon *et al.*, 1986). A peritoneal factor inhibiting ovum pick-up was demonstrated in women with endometriosis by Suginami *et al.* (1986). Altered tubal transport of the fertilized ovum may be related to an increased concentration of prostaglandins in the peritoneal fluid, although data on the concentration of prostaglandins is conflicting. However, experimental modification of tubal transport by prostaglandins has not been successful, and the early entry of the embryo

into the uterus as a cause of infertility is not supported by the clinical success of IVF.

The peritoneal fluid from women with endometriosis has been shown to have an adverse effect on spermatozoa and on pre-implantation embryos *in vitro*. This has been related either to an increased number of peritoneal macrophages in an advanced state of activation, or an effect of their secretory products such as interleukin-1 (Halme *et al.*, 1984; Haney *et al.*, 1981). It has also been suggested that embryo development in the fallopian tube may be adversely affected by the increased capability of these macrophages to secrete interleukin-1 at the time of fertilization and early cleavage. On the other hand, normal motile spermatozoa have been recovered from peritoneal fluid 4 hours after insemination in women with endometriosis (Stone & Himsl, 1986), and peritoneal fluid and macrophage supernatants from such women were not embryotoxic in an *in vitro* mouse system (Awadalla *et al.*, 1987).

Autoimmunity

An autoimmune response to ectopic endometrium has also been postulated as a cause of implantation failure, but the level of endometrial autoantibodies is not elevated in women with mild endometriosis (Halme & Mathur, 1987), and the hypothesis is not supported by the clinical results from IVF programmes which show no difference in implantation failure between women with endometriosis and those with tubal infertility.

Although a high spontaneous abortion rate ranging from 30–50% has been reported in women with endometriosis, FitzSimmons *et al.* (1987) found no difference in the rates in women with and without endometriosis, and suggested that the apparent improvement in outcome following therapy could be related to selection bias.

Conclusion

Despite considerable research and discussion, no cause has emerged to explain the diminished fertility of women with endometriosis, and treatment of this condition will continue to be controversial. Most studies show little benefit from treating mild disease, and extensive endometriosis remains resistant to medical or surgical therapy.

3.2 THE NORMAL PELVIC PERITONEUM
Freddy Cornillie

The normal and pathological fine structure of the human peritoneum is poorly understood. Nevertheless it is generally accepted that regurgitated menstrual elements may implant on the peritoneal surface or stimulate peritoneal metaplasia. Study of the peritoneum is therefore of utmost importance to the understanding of the pathogenesis of pelvic endometriosis.

The normal pelvic peritoneum is basically composed of three layers: the mesothelial lining, a basement membrane and the submesothelial connective tissue layer. Each layer may play a part in the normal, and abnormal, functioning of the pelvic peritoneum.

The Mesothelial Lining

The mesothelial lining is composed of flattened squamous cells covering the surface of the pelvic peritoneum. Scanning electron microscopy has shown microvilli on the cell surface bordering the peritoneal cavity, which appear to be more numerous on the peripheral cell margins adjacent to the intercellular junctions (Fig. 3.2.1a). Occasionally the mesothelial cells bear a single cilium, but ciliated cells, such as are found in the fallopian tube, and in eutopic and ectopic endometrium, are not seen. The nucleus occupies a central position and the cell bulges into the peritoneal cavity. Thus the apical surface of the mesothelium is in contact with the peritoneal fluid (Fig. 3.2.1b), whilst the basal region of the cell rests on the basement membrane. This cellular polarity is indicative of cells involved in the secretion or resorption of substances in either direction, and suggests that the mesothelial lining cells are involved in the transport of substances into and away from the peritoneal cavity.

Narrow invaginations of the mesothelial lining create a ruffled peritoneal substructure which is not visible at laparoscopy. Although these structures may resemble glandular orifices, they have no secretory function and represent only peritoneal microfolds (Fig. 3.2.1c).

The use of transmission electron microscopy has enabled detailed examination of the subcellular organization of the mesothelial cells. The cell organelles are distributed throughout the central perinuclear and peripheral cytoplasmic zones, and the frequent occurrence of mitochondria and pinocytic vesicles (Fig. 3.2.1d) indicates that the cells are involved in active secretion and resorption. The mitochondria yield the adenosine triphosphate (ATP) necessary to generate energy for such active cytoplasmic processes as endocytosis and pinocytosis.

Endocytotic and pinocytotic vesicles shuttle in both directions across the mesothelial lining from one cell pole to the other. The former transport specific ligands

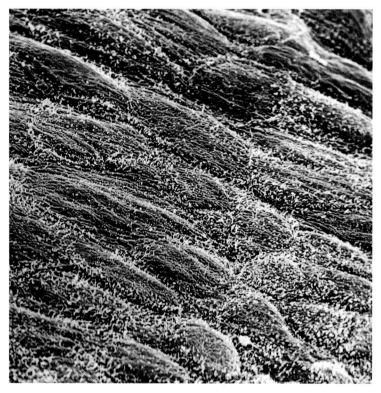

Fig. 3.2.1a–d The mesothelial lining.
a Scanning electronmicrograph (SEM) showing the ultrastructure of the surface of the normal peritoneum. Numerous microvilli are present on the peripheral margins of the mesothelial cells (×2000).

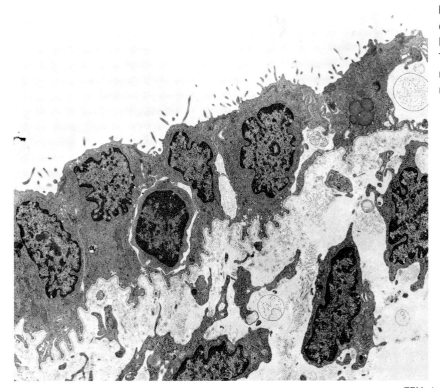

b Transmission electronmicrograph (TEM) of the ultrastructure of the mesothelial lining and the subjacent connective tissue. The mesothelial cells rest on a basement membrane. A lymphocyte is seen within the mesothelial lining ($\times$5400).

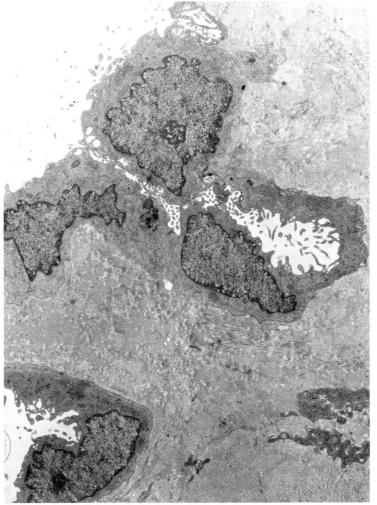

c TEM showing that microfolds of the peritoneal surface may resemble glandular structures but lack any obvious secretory activity ($\times$5400).

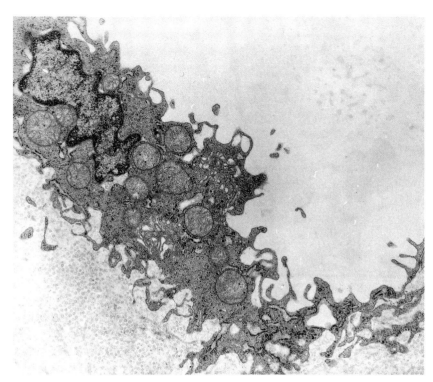

Fig. 3.2.1 continued.

d TEM of the mesothelial cells. There are numerous mitochondria and transcellular vesicular channels in the lateral cytoplasm of the mesothelial cells (×14,000).

(receptor-mediated endocytosis) while the latter transport only fluid and small solutes. As a result, secondary lysosomes are found in many cells of the peritoneal lining. Large lysosomes containing engulfed foreign particles or damaged cells are, however, absent from the mesothelium, indicating that there is no active intracellular defence mechanism against foreign body or cell attack. The mesothelial lining therefore represents a selective sieve-barrier between the peritoneal tissue and the peritoneal cavity.

The Basement Membrane

The basement membrane is a continuous amorphous layer secreted by the mesothelial cells. Although its ultrastructure resembles the epithelial basement membrane in many other tissues, its biochemical composition has not been investigated. The basement membrane does not prevent the migration of blood-borne cells from the submesothelial connective tissue into the mesothelial lining and the peritoneal cavity (Fig. 3.2.2).

The Submesothelial Connective Tissue

The fine structure of the submesothelial connective tissue may show various focal patterns, with areas of loose organization interspersed with fibrous connective tissue and thick collagen bundles. This collagen, together with other extracellular matrix components, is secreted by the numerous fibroblasts in this tissue.

Focal oedema formation which may be observed particularly around the microvasculature within the loose connective tissue areas is probably controlled by these microvessels. It has been shown that the endothelial cells of the venules contain histamine receptors, and that histamine increases their permeability by opening the endothelial intercellular junctions. In addition, granulated mast cells containing histamine are a common finding (Fig. 3.2.3).

Pigment-laden cells are not found in the peritoneum and the normal peritoneal tint is produced by extension of the local microvasculature and/or oedema formation, the pink areas having a more extensive blood supply. Occasionally, dilatation of microvessels and extravasation of blood into the submesothelial connective tissues are seen. These focal abnormalities may be visible during laparoscopy as small reddish spots, representing focal microhaemorrhages, on the peritoneum. Although these spots may be suspected as evidence of endometriosis, they do not usually contain any endometriotic tissue (Brosens & Cornillie, 1987).

The deeper layers of the submesothelial connective tissue of the uterovesical fold and the uterosacral ligaments contain smooth muscle cells. Contraction of these cells may diminish the blood flow through the superficial tissues and may thus influence their function.

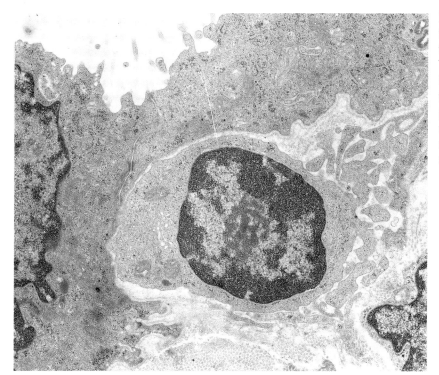

Fig. 3.2.2 Migration of lymphocytes from the submesothelial connective tissue into the peritoneal fluid.
TEM of peritoneal surface showing lymphocytes migrating from the peritoneal tissue into the peritoneal fluid. During this process the basement membrane of the mesothelium is disrupted and the mesothelial intercellular junctions are opened (×14,000).

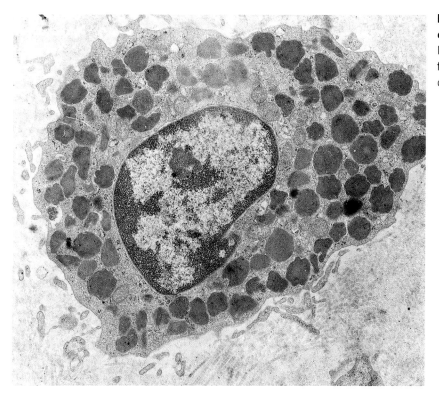

Fig. 3.2.3 Mast cell in submesothelial connective tissue.
Mast cells containing typical granules are frequently seen in the submesothelial connective tissue (×14,000).

Conclusion

The pelvic peritoneum thus forms an active tissue barrier covering a large surface area. The interaction between peritoneum and peritoneal fluid is poorly understood however, and needs extensive investigation in both normal and abnormal conditions.

In addition, there is currently no conclusive information as to whether the peritoneal tissues undergo morphological or functional changes during the menstrual cycle and particularly during menstruation.

3.3 PERITONEAL ENDOMETRIOSIS
Freddy Cornillie

The structure of peritoneal endometriotic lesions depends on their site, and the evolution of the disease may be regulated by the local conditions. Recent attention has been focused on the subtle clinical appearance of early endometriosis, which presents as peritoneal defects, and on microscopic implants, which are invisible at laparoscopy (Vasquez *et al.*, 1984; Jansen & Russell, 1986; Stripling *et al.*, 1988).

At present there is no morphological evidence that foreign cells, including endometrial cells, implant on the mesothelium, and if the implantation of endometrial cells is the earliest event in the pathogenesis of endometriosis, more detailed studies are required. However, the implantation of single cells or small groups of cells is difficult to detect, even by scanning electron microscopy. Also, as implantation may occur before the onset of symptomatic disease, the initial events may be missed.

Laparoscopic Evaluation of Peritoneal Endometriosis

The clinical diagnosis of endometriosis is made by laparoscopy, and confirmed by the presence of endometriotic tissue (ectopic glands and stroma) on histological examination of biopsy specimens.

As well as confirming the diagnosis, there are at least two other reasons for biopsying endometriotic implants found at laparoscopy.

1. The degree of cellular differentiation of the implant, which reflects its hormone dependency, can be assessed (Schweppe & Wynn, 1984). Hormone therapy should be more effective for well differentiated implants.

2. Post-treatment biopsies can be studied to evaluate the effect of medical therapy (Cornillie *et al.*, 1985). Treatments, including danazol, dydrogesterone, or gonadotrophin releasing hormone (GnRH) agonists do not eliminate the implants but, in some cases, produce marked involution together with an increase in the number of lysosomes. Such changes are considered to be satisfactory responses to therapy.

The laparoscopic diagnosis of endometriosis is usually based on the recognition of ectopic implants of endometrial tissue and is evaluated, not on its activity, but on its visible sequelae such as fibrosis, pigmentation, adhesion formation, and the presence of an endometrioma. Various classifications have been proposed on the basis of the presence and extent of these sequelae and have been extensively used for comparing the results of surgical treatment, but their value in pathophysiological studies and in the evaluation of medical therapy has been questioned (Brosens *et al.*, 1987; Evers, 1987).

Three different types of peritoneal implant can be distinguished and each may represent different stages in the development of endometriosis.

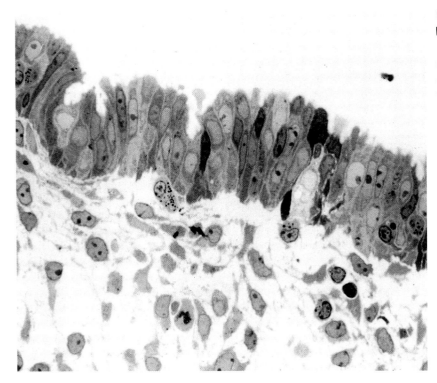

Fig. 3.3.1 Epithelial plaque-type implant.
Plaque-type endometriotic implant which is composed of endometrial surface epithelium and stroma. Note the presence of so-called endometrial granulocytes within the subepithelial stroma (×800).

The Epithelial Plaque-Type Implant

The epithelial plaque-type implant which is usually well differentiated and active, is unpigmented, and therefore usually invisible at laparoscopy. Using scanning electron microscopy, Murphy *et al.* (1986), found these lesions in 25% of biopsies taken from apparently normal areas of the peritoneum of patients with endometriosis, where the pelvic peritoneum appeared to be replaced by endometrial epithelium (Fig. 3.3.1). The lesions may be considered to be an intraperitoneal endometriosis as it is in contact with the peritoneal cavity, and secretory products of the endometriotic epithelium can pass into the peritoneal fluid.

The Vesicular-Type Implant

The vesicular-type implant presents with single or multiple, clear or pigmented blisters, which are less than 5 mm in diameter at laparoscopy. Sometimes the implant may be red in colour and there is increased vascularization of the surrounding peritoneum. Biopsies studied by scanning electron microscopy and histological techniques have shown that these vesicles contain active endometriotic implants in the form of either polypoid structures or cystically dilated glands (Cornillie *et al.*, 1986).

The polypoid form contains polyps of glandular endometriotic cells arising in the subjacent peritoneal tissue (Fig. 3.3.2a). Serial sectioning of these implants has shown that the polyps are composed of an outer layer of endometrial epithelium surrounding a central core of well differentiated and highly vascularized stroma (Fig. 3.3.2b). *In vivo*, these are probably suspended within a fluid-filled vesicle whose wall is derived from the peritoneal mesothelium, which flattens and stretches as the vesicle forms (Fig. 3.3.2c). This vesicular wall usually ruptures whilst the biopsy is being taken and its absence from biopsy specimens should therefore be considered as an artefact.

Formation of the vesicle is probably triggered by the secretion of osmotically active compounds, including glycoproteins, by the endometrial epithelium, which creates a concentration gradient between the active implant and the surrounding tissues and peritoneal fluid. Osmotic uptake of water into the space around the implant results in the formation of a fluid-filled vesicle whose size depends on the osmotic pressure and hence the secretory activity of the endometrial implant within. Ultimately the fluid pressure in the vesicle probably reaches a critical level and causes the wall to rupture, thereby releasing the vesicular contents into the peritoneal cavity and transforming the subperitoneal polypoid form of vesicular implant into an intraperitoneal lesion.

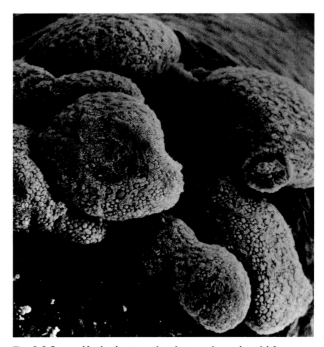

Fig. 3.3.2a–c Vesicular-type implant – the polypoid form.
a SEM of a polypoid endometriotic lesion which is composed of several polyps (×220).

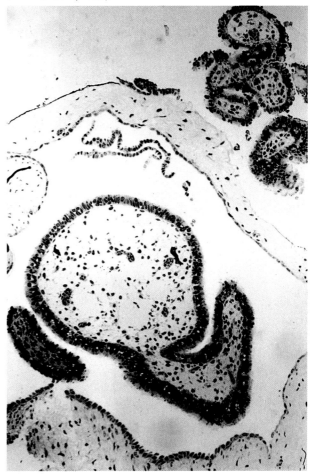

b Each polyp is covered with endometrial surface epithelium. Note also the presence of endometriotic tissue beneath (×235).

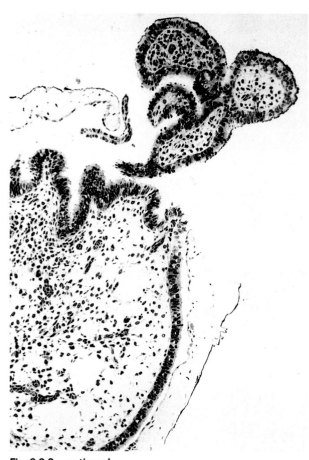

Vesicles which contain one or more cystically dilated glands (Fig. 3.3.3a) differ morphologically from the polypoid form although the foci of endometrial epithelia are similarly located in the submesothelium. The active endometrial cells secrete substances into the lumina of the glands (Fig. 3.3.3b) leading to an increasing concentration of osmotically active compounds. This induces water retention and dilatation of the gland, which causes the glandular epithelium to flatten whilst still retaining its secretory activity (Fig. 3.3.3c). As the cystically dilated gland enlarges, a vesicle wall forms from the distorted mesothelium and submesothelial connective tissues. This wall eventually undergoes pressure necrosis and may rupture.

The histology and ultrastructure of vesicular-type lesions suggests that this 'so-called' minimal endometriosis is, in fact, an early and very active stage of the disease.

Fig. 3.3.2 continued.
c The peritoneal mesothelium has ruptured. The polyps and the submesothelial part of the implant contain oedematous and well-vascularized stroma (×235).

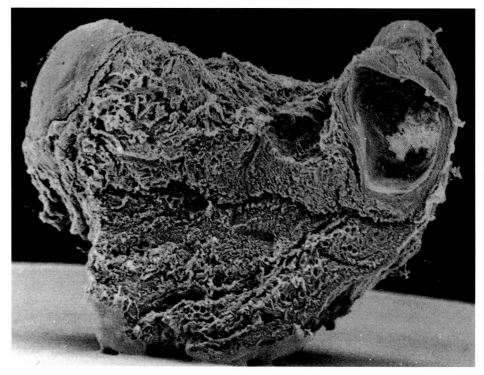

Fig. 3.3.3a–c Vesicular-type implant – the cystically dilated gland form.
a An endometriotic implant with a large, cystically dilated gland. The peritoneal surface at this area bulges into the peritoneal cavity (×40).

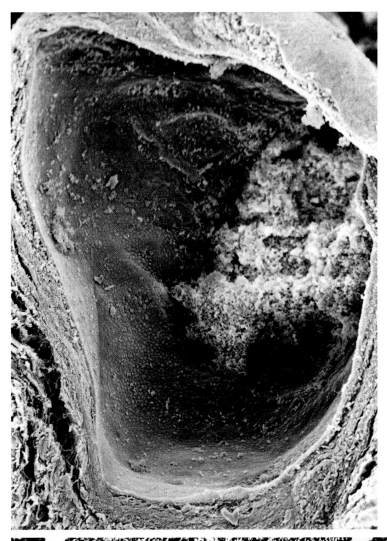

b An intraluminal view of the cystic gland shows that secretory substances have accumulated within it (×150).

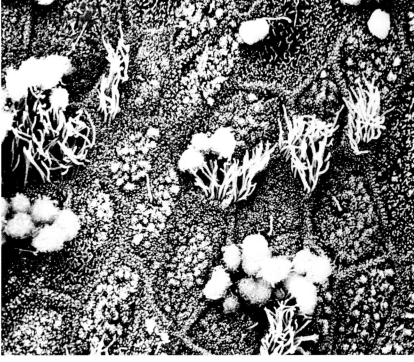

c SEM showing the substructure of the apical cell region of the epithelial cells lining the cystic gland. Secretory granules accumulate within the lumen. Note also the prominent cell junctions and their ciliated cells (×3000).

Pigmented Plaques

Pigmented plaques form the typical 'powder-burn' dark blue lesions that are easily seen on the pelvic peritoneum at laparoscopy. Histopathological studies of these lesions show the remnants of endometriotic tissue, which are mainly inactive, embedded in pigment-laden connective tissue areas (Fig. 3.3.4).

These implants must be differentiated from other peritoneal lesions such as inflammatory or infectious lesions, foreign body reactions, or fibrous deposits. Small subperitoneal dilated vessels or haemorrhages may also mimic endometriosis.

Activity of Peritoneal Implants of Endometriosis

Endometriotic implants have been shown to have steroid receptors but these are less numerous than in eutopic endometrium; a variable degree of steroid responsiveness is seen in the implant during the menstrual cycle depending on its characteristics (Nieminen, 1962).
1. Cyclical changes corresponding with those of the endometrium, including late secretory changes and menstrual bleeding are seen in free-growing implants. These have a polypoid or cauliflower structure, and grow along the surface. They are characterized by a surface epithelium supported by endometrial stroma.
2. The enclosed implant rarely shows cyclical changes during the menstrual cycle, and late secretory changes and menstrual bleeding do not occur. These implants have no surface epithelium and are located within tissue or are part of a free-growing lesion. They may also present as wedge-like extensions of stroma deep in tissues, connecting one lesion with another. During the menstrual cycle, capillary and venous dilatation occur, but there is no arterial necrosis or bleeding at the time of menstruation.

The healed lesion is characterized by cystically enlarged glands with a thin glandular epithelium supported by small, fusiform stromal cells and surrounded by connective tissue.

These observations by Nieminen support the view that the hormonal response in peritoneal endometriosis may depend on the type of implant. The vesicular implant can respond fully to the ovarian steroids, frequently has a haemorrhagic appearance, and biopsies almost always show the presence of endometrial tissue.

The so-called 'typical peritoneal lesion' is likely to represent different stages of an enclosed lesion. An active enclosed lesion may become a healed inactive lesion depending on the regression of the stromal component, and the increase in connective tissue and fibrosis. As flattening and involutionary changes in the glandular epithelium are characteristic of a healed lesion, it is not surprising that endometrial tissue is not often found in them.

The Extent of Peritoneal Endometriosis

Mild endometriosis as defined by The American Fertility Society classification (1985) is not confined to a homogeneous group of women with minimal disease, but ranges from a pelvis full of small, active but almost

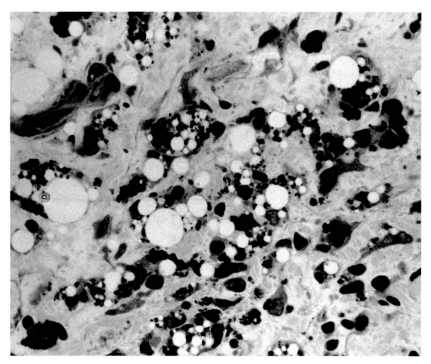

Fig. 3.3.4 'Powder-burn' lesion.
'Powder-burn' lesion showing the submesothelial connective tissue with pigment-laden phagocytes. Sometimes there are no endometrial glands and stroma (×800).

invisible implants, to the presence of a single fibrotic inactive implant. Studies on the pathophysiology and the clinical significance of mild endometriosis may differ greatly with regard to the extent and activity of peritoneal endometriosis and may yield different results.

Clinical studies of the effect of medical therapy may also be misleading when the peritoneal endometriosis is evaluated before and after suppressive therapy which may mask the small active implant by resorption of its secretory and haemorrhagic products. In the absence of a specific marker for active peritoneal endometriosis,

it is important to be aware of the limitations of laparoscopic evaluation.

Conclusion

To learn more about the pathophysiology and evolution of this enigmatic disease, attention should be focused on the early and superficial implants. These active lesions may eventually transform into typical pigmented plaques, accompanied by intermittent bleeding, pigment formation and, ultimately, fibrotic fibrosis.

3.4 OVARIAN ENDOMETRIOSIS

In more advanced stages of endometriosis, the tubes, ovaries and surrounding structures may become distorted. The type and the extent of the lesion influence the choice of treatment. Ovarian endometriosis presents as superficial haemorrhagic lesions or, in the more severe forms, as haemorrhagic cysts.

Superficial Lesions

The superficial lesions of ovarian endometriosis are usually found on the lateral surface of the ovary (Fig. 3.4.1) and have a strong tendency to form adhesions with similar lesions on the peritoneum of the broad ligament or to other adjacent organs including the omentum, bowel and fallopian tube.

Endometrioma

The term 'chocolate cyst' was applied by Sampson (1921) to describe the endometrial cyst of the ovary. The term is, however, purely descriptive and can be

misleading if only the chocolate-coloured contents of the cyst are noted, as haemorrhagic dysfunctional cysts are frequently encountered in ovarian endometriosis, postoperative ovarian adhesive disease or in the presence of the sequelae of pelvic inflammatory disease. Features indicative of endometriosis are the site of the cyst, the presence of adhesions and the formation of a puckered scar (Fig. 3.4.2). However, not infrequently an endometriotic cyst can have a smooth surface with few adhesions, or it may occur in combination with a haemorrhagic dysfunctional cyst; in such cases, the macroscopic diagnosis of its endometrial origin can be difficult or impossible.

Histopathology

There is considerable variation in the pattern of ovarian endometriosis.

1. The endometrial cyst may be lined by free endometrial tissue that cannot be distinguished histologically and functionally from eutopic endometrium. Such implants can cover the inner surface of a small cavity in the ovary, such as a corpus fibrosum. Nieminen (1962), has shown

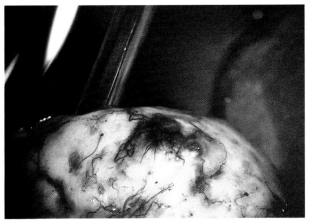

Fig. 3.4.1 Ovarian endometriosis.
Endometriosis on the surface of the ovary presenting as a free-growing haemorrhagic lesion.

that the vascularization of free-growing endometriosis fully corresponds with the cyclical changes in the endometrial vasculature, including the degeneration and necrosis leading to menstrual bleeding.

2. Ovarian endometriosis may also produce enclosed lesions, in which the cavity is covered with fibrotic tissue and glandular epithelium, and sparsely surrounded by stroma, with glandular structures in the fibrotic wall of the cyst. The cyclical changes of these enclosed lesions are less significant than those in the free-growing lesions and late secretory changes and menstrual bleeding are absent. The haemorrhagic content of these cysts probably originates from persisting small implants of free endometriosis or congested vessels at the hilus of the ovary. Occasionally a haemorrhagic corpus luteum can be associated with an endometrial cyst.

Hughesdon (1957), has pointed out that the internal surface of a chocolate cyst is really the external surface of the ovary; the ovarian cortex is identifiable by the

presence of primordial follicles. These cysts cannot be mobilized from their fixed position in the ovarian fossa or on the broad ligament without their rupture and subsequent spillage of contents.

Rationale for Surgical Treatment in Infertility

Surgery is necessary for the mechanical sequelae of endometriosis. Gordts *et al.* (1984) found that the cumulative pregnancy rate following microsurgery in patients with severe endometriosis was the same as in patients with mild endometriosis.

The concept of microscopic implants of endometriosis suggests that surgical treatment of visible endometriosis is, in reality, a debulking procedure. Postoperative adhesion formation however is common after extensive pelvic surgery and is a major indication for repeat surgery. Although laparoscopic laser techniques using carbon dioxide or argon laser (see page 5.18) provide precise and accurate methods of surgical treatment, microscopic implants cannot always be identified even with the magnification provided by the laparoscope; the area of implantation can however be suspected by the presence of a pattern of increased fine vasculature, minute adhesion formation or peritoneal defects. Photocoagulation by argon laser is a particularly elegant technique for destroying the vascular network and the active, highly vascularized peritoneal implant.

At present little data are available to compare the efficacy of the different surgical techniques by evaluating the pregnancy rates and the recurrence, persistence or evolution of the endometriosis.

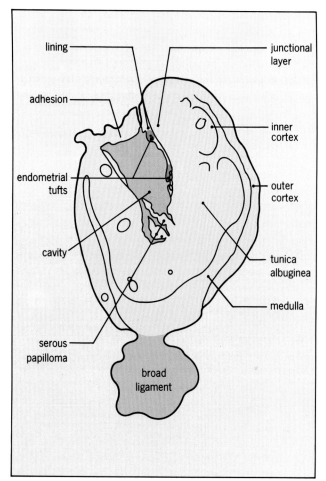

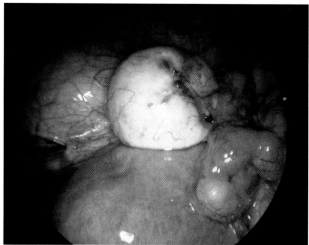

Fig. 3.4.2a & b Ovarian endometriosis.
a The structure of an ovarian endometrioma – a diagrammatic representation. The inside of the 'chocolate cyst' is the outside of the ovarian cortex. (From Hughesdon, 1957.)

b Typical appearance of an ovarian endometrioma: implantation on the lateral side of the ovary associated with puckering and pigmented scar formation.

Ovarioscopy

Conservative ovarian surgery is a major cause of ovarian adhesive disease, and recurrent cyst formation is the most common indication for a second operative procedure on the ovary. Ovarioscopy has been developed to gain access to the ovarian cyst at the time of diagnostic or operative laparoscopy. This endoscopic approach to the cyst is preceded by a careful clinical, sonar, laboratory and laparoscopic evaluation. Factors influencing the selection of cases for intra-ovarian surgery are the age of the patient, her ovulatory status, a history of endometriosis, and the characteristics of the cyst and its contents.

Technique

Ovarioscopy is based on the double optic laparoscopic technique developed for salpingoscopy (see page 4.18). The instruments consist of a 2.6 mm endoscope in a

5 mm operating sheath with a groove that allows the passage of an infusion, and small instruments such as biopsy forceps and a laser fibre (Fig. 3.4.3).

Following inspection with an operating laparoscope so that the optimal site of entry can be identified, the cyst is punctured and the fluid aspirated for cytological examination.

The ovarioscope is then introduced into the cyst through the small puncture hole, a saline infusion is allowed to run freely to wash out and distend the cyst, and the wall is inspected in detail. Biopsies can be taken under direct vision for histopathological study. Several different types of cyst can be identified.

Functional Cysts

The wall of a follicular cyst is characterized by a smooth and undulating surface overlying a fine, regular network of small vessels (Fig. 3.4.4). The corpus luteum cyst is

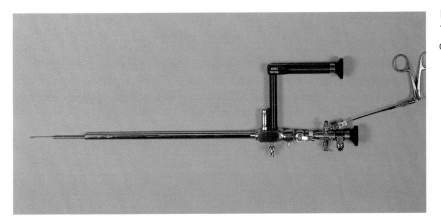

Fig. 3.4.3 The ovarioscope.
The ovarioscope with biopsy forceps in the operating channel of the laparoscope.

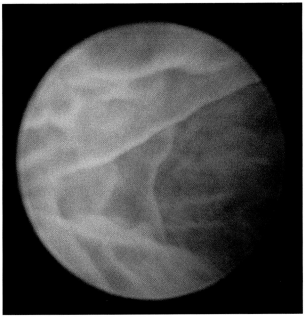

Fig. 3.4.4 Follicular cyst.
The follicular cyst has a smooth undulating surface.

identified by the presence of luteinized areas, which may involve only part of the cyst. The vascular network is prominent and foci of extravasation can be identified (Fig. 3.4.5). The cyst cavity may be partially occluded by fibrin fibres.

Ovarian Endometriotic Cyst

The wall of an ovarian endometrioma can present a wide variety of appearances. Dark fibrotic areas with haemosiderin pigmentation but little superficial vascularization alternate with areas which are highly vascularized and have foci of bleeding. The vessels in these areas are often congested and protrude onto the surface as small haemorrhoids, and tend to be larger and more congested at the hilus of the ovary. Occasionally, a haemorrhagic corpus luteum cyst can be identified within the endometrioma.

It is suggested that the haemorrhagic content of many 'chocolate cysts' may originate from chronic focal bleeding from congested blood vessels rather than from endometrial shedding. Much of the wall of an endometrioma is composed of fibrotic and reactive tissue lined with endometrial cells, which show a poor cyclical response during the menstrual cycle and hormonal therapy (Cornillie *et al.*, 1985). Clinically, ovarian endometrial tissue is resistant to medical therapy. The fibrotic areas in ovarian endometriosis with enclosed endometrium are therefore unlikely to be the site of menstrual bleeding, and the bleeding is more likely to originate from small areas such as the sites of congested vessels at the hilus of the ovary or some areas with 'free' endometriosis. These areas can be identified at ovarioscopy by the presence of superficial vascularization.

Intra-Ovarian Argon Laser Therapy

If the haemorrhagic content of ovarian endometriomata is due to chronic focal bleeding, as hypothesized above, such lesions that originate from focal bleeding points can be treated by selective coagulation of the haemorrhagic areas with argon laser (Fig. 3.4.6). Ovarioscopy is performed, the cavity is flushed with saline, and an argon laser fibre is threaded through the groove in the sheath to coagulate the wall of the cyst under direct vision. The argon laser is particularly useful for this purpose because of its selective absorption by haemopigments. The depth of penetration of the laser energy does not exceed 0.8 mm and damage to surrounding healthy ovarian tissue can therefore be avoided.

Ovarioscopy is likely to be particularly useful in patients with so-called recurrent endometriosis after ovarian surgery. In many of these patients, the recurrence of the cyst is caused by postoperative adhesive disease of the ovary, which is frequently associated with dysfunctional, haemorrhagic and non-haemorrhagic cyst formation. Accurate diagnosis of the nature of the cyst at second-look laparoscopy with ovarioscopy can therefore avoid the performance of an unnecessary laparotomy.

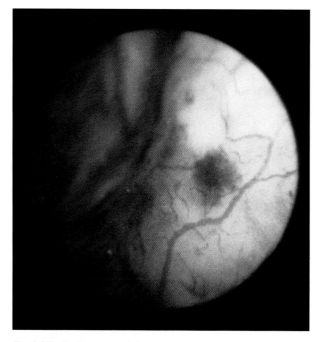

Fig. 3.4.5 Cystic corpus luteum.
Luteinization and a small haemorrhagic area can be seen in this cystic corpus luteum.

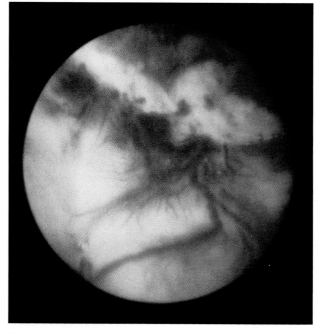

Fig. 3.4.6 Congested vessels in a haemorrhagic corpus luteum.

REFERENCES

The American Fertility Society. (1985) Revised American Fertility Society classification of endometriosis. *Fertility and Sterility*, **43**, 351–352.

Awadalla, S.G., Friedman, C.I., Haq, A.U., Roh, S.I., Chin, N.O.W. & Kim, M.H. (1987) Local peritoneal factors: their role in infertility associated with endometriosis. *American Journal of Obstetrics and Gynecology*, **157**, 1207–1214.

Brosens, I. & Cornillie, F. (1987) Peritoneal endometriosis. Morphological basis of the laparoscopic diagnosis. In: *Endometriosis. Contributions to Gynecology and Obstetrics*. Volume 16. Edited by M. Bruhat & M. Canis. pp.125–137.

Brosens, I., Cornillie, F. & Vasquez, G. (1987) Etiology and pathophysiology of endometriosis. In: *Gonadotrophin down-regulation in gynaecological practice*. Edited by R. Rolland, D.R. Chada & W.N.P. Willemsen. *Progress in Clinical and Biological Research*, **225**, 81–102.

Cornillie, F., Vasquez, G. & Brosens, I. (1985) The response of human endometriotic implants to the anti-progesterone steroid R 2323: a histologic and ultrastructural study. *Pathology, Research and Practice*, **180**, 647–655.

Cornillie, F., Brosens, I., Vasquez, G. & Riphagen, I. (1986) Histologic and ultrastructural changes in human endometriotic implants treated with the antiprogesterone steroid ethylnorgestrienone (Gestrinone) during 2 months. *International Journal of Gynecological Pathology*, **5**, 95–109.

Doody, M.C., Gibbons, W.E. & Buttram, J.C.Jr. (1988) Linear regression analysis of ultrasound follicular growth series: evidence for an abnormality of follicular growth in endometriosis patients. *Fertility and Sterility*, **49**, 47–51.

Evers, J.L.H. (1987) The second-look laparoscopy for evaluation of the result of medical treatment of endometriosis should not be performed during ovarian suppression. *Fertility and Sterility*, **47**, 696–698.

FitzSimmons, J., Stahl, R., Gocial, B. & Shapiro, S.S. (1987) Spontaneous abortion and endometriosis. *Fertility and Sterility*, **42**, 696–698.

Gordts, S., Boeckx, W. & Brosens, I. (1984) Microsurgery of endometriosis in infertile patients. *Fertility and Sterility*, **42**, 520–525.

Halme, J., Becker, S. & Wing, R. (1984) Accentuated cyclic activation of peritoneal macrophages in patients with endometriosis. *American Journal of Obstetrics and Gynecology*, **148**, 85–90.

Halme, J. & Mathur, S. (1987) Local autoimmunity in mild endometriosis. *International Journal of Fertility*, **32**, 309–311.

Hammond, M.G., Jordan, S. & Sloan, C.S. (1986) Factors affecting pregnancy rates in a donor insemination program using frozen semen. *American Journal of Obstetrics and Gynecology*, **155**, 480–485.

Haney, A.F., Muscato, J.J. & Weinberg, J.B. (1981) Peritoneal fluid cell populations in infertility patients. *Fertility and Sterility*, **35**, 696–698.

Hughesdon, P.E. (1957) The structure of endometrial cysts of the ovary. *The Journal of Obstetrics and Gynaecology of the British Empire*, **64**, 481–487.

Jansen, R.P.S. (1986) Minimal endometriosis and reduced fecundibility: prospective evidence from an artificial insemination by donor program. *Fertility and Sterility*, **46**, 141–143.

Jansen, R. & Russell, P. (1986) Nonpigmented endometriosis: clinical, laparoscopic and pathologic definitions. *American Journal of Obstetrics and Gynecology*, **155**, 1154–1159.

Kauppila, A., Rajaniemi, H. & Roennberg, L. (1982) Low LH (hCG) receptor concentration in ovarian follicles in endometriosis. *Acta Obstetrica et Gynecologica Scandinavica*, **61**, 81–83.

Murphy, A., Green, W., Bobbie, D., dela Cruz, Z. & Rock, J. (1986) Unsuspected endometriosis documented by scanning electron microscopy in visually normal peritoneum. *Fertility and Sterility*, **46**, 522–524.

Nieminen, V. (1962) Studies on the vascular pattern of ectopic endometrium with special reference to cyclic changes. *Acta Obstetrica et Gynecologica Scandinavica*, **41** (Suppl. 3), 1–82.

Roennberg, L., Kauppila, A. & Rajaniemi, H. (1984) Luteinizing hormone receptor disorder in endometriosis. *Fertility and Sterility*, **42**, 64–68.

Sampson, J.A. (1921) Perforating haemorrhagic (chocolate) cysts of the ovary: their importance and especially their relation to pelvic adenomas of endometrial type (adenomyoma of the uterus, rectovaginal septum, sigmoid, etc.) *Archives of Surgery*, **3**, 245–323.

Schenken, R. & Asch, R. (1980) Surgical induction of endometriosis in the rabbit: effects on fertility and concentrations of peritoneal fluid prostaglandins. *Fertility and Sterility*, **34**, 581–587.

Schweppe, K. & Wynn, R. (1984) Endocrine dependency of endometriosis: an ultrastructural study. *European Journal of Obstetrics and Gynecology and Reproductive Biology*, **17**, 173–208.

Stone, S.C. & Himsl, K. (1986) Peritoneal recovery of motile and nonmotile sperm in the presence of endometriosis. *Fertility and Sterility*, **46**, 338–339.

Stripling, M., Martin, D., Chatman, D., Vander Zwaag, R. & Poston, W. (1988) Subtle appearance of pelvic endometriosis. *Fertility and Sterility*, **49**, 427–431.

Suginami, H., Yano, K., Watanabe, K. & Matsuura, S. (1986) A factor inhibiting ovum capture by the oviductal fimbriae. *Fertility and Sterility*, **46**, 1140–1146.

Thomas, E.J. & Cooke, I.D. (1987) Successful treatment of asymptomatic endometriosis: Does it benefit infertile women? *British Medical Journal*, **294**, 1117–1119.

Thomas, E.J., Lenton, E.A. & Cooke, I.D. (1986) Follicle growth patterns and endocrinological abnormalities in infertile women with minor degrees of endometriosis. *British Journal of Obstetrics and Gynaecology*, **93**, 852–858.

Vasquez, G., Cornillie, F. & Brosens, I. (1984) Peritoneal endometriosis: scanning electron microscopy and histology of minimal pelvic endometriotic lesions. *Fertility and Sterility*, **42**, 696–703.

Vernon, M., Beard, J., Graves, J. & Wilson, E. (1986) Classification of endometriotic implants by morphologic appearance and capacity to synthesize prostaglandin F. *Fertility and Sterility*, **46**, 801–806.

4 **INVESTIGATION OF TUBAL INFERTILITY**

4.1 INTRODUCTION

When investigating the female genital tract in infertility, a multidisciplinary approach should be adopted.

A detailed clinical history together with a complete physical examination is always necessary. Special attention should be paid to lower abdominal pain or dyspareunia, and any evidence of pelvic tenderness, past or present, should alert the physician to the possibility of pelvic inflammatory disease. The importance of an accurate history was demonstrated by Cumming and Taylor (1979), whose laparoscopic studies showed that 75% of women with a suggestive history, but only 24% of those with a non-contributory history, had demonstrable pelvic pathology. In addition, Westrom and Märdh (1980), have stressed that a history of upper genital tract infection may indicate the presence of tubal obstruction; 11.4% of women with a history of one attack of salpingitis were found to have blocked tubes, but after two and three attacks this figure rose to 23.1% and 54.3%, respectively. These investigators also stressed the high incidence of infection with *Chlamydia trachomatis* and suggested that this should always be excluded before performing hysterosalpingography.

Hysterosalpingography vs Laparoscopy

Radiological studies complement endoscopic investigations as each provides information, albeit with a varying degree of accuracy, about one or more segments of the oviduct, and each can also be used to confirm the findings of the other.

There are considerable discrepancies between the findings at hysterosalpingography and laparoscopy in the presence of peritubal adhesions or endometriosis. In a series of 500 women investigated by Donnez *et al.* (1982), these techniques gave comparable information regarding tubal patency in 90% of cases. However conglutination of the fimbriae was detected twice as often by laparoscopy than by hysterosalpingography, which also detected only 68% of peritubal adhesions. Failure to detect and treat such lesions leads to continued infertility, although occasionally conception does occur in women who have such extensive pelvic disease that the likelihood appears remote.

Hysterosalpingography and Laparoscopy vs Salpingoscopy

Although the mucosal folds can be outlined by hysterosalpingography, the correlation between radiological studies and endoscopy in the assessment of the tubal mucosa is poor. The importance of salpingoscopy was demonstrated by Henry-Suchet *et al.* (1984), who examined 231 tubes during tubal microsurgery and found that the lesions in the ampulla differed from those predicted by hysterosalpingography in a significant number of cases (Fig. 4.1.1). Abnormal tubal mucosa at hysterosalpingography was confirmed by salpingoscopy in only 38% of cases. Conversely, a normal tubal mucosa at hysterosalpingography was confirmed in 58% of cases, but the remainder showed lesions such as areas of flattened mucosa and adhesions which had not been detected radiologically.

Brosens and Vasquez (1976), used scanning electron microscopy on microbiopsy specimens to demonstrate that, in infertile patients with apparently normal tubes on hysterosalpingography and laparoscopy, there were lesions of the mucosa such as flattening of the folds, loss of cilia and alteration of the cilial pattern. They considered these lesions to be a major cause of infertility and of failure of tubal reconstructive surgery.

The authors have also found discrepancies between the findings of laparoscopy and salpingoscopy. In distal tubal blockage, the mucosa was normal in 62% of cases, whereas when the tubes were patent it was abnormal in 5%. This suggests that failure to perform salpingoscopy during the investigation of infertility could lead to an inaccurate assessment of tubal morphology. This is of particular importance when gamete intrafallopian transfer (GIFT) is being considered because the gametes may be transferred into a tube which, although normal by the standard criteria, may possess mucosal abnormalities which would interfere with their transport.

Multidisciplinary investigation requires skill and patience; the techniques must be taught with care and their application may not be within the scope of every clinician.

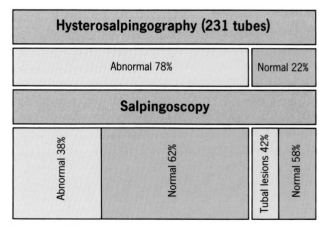

Fig. 4.1.1 Salpingoscopy vs hysterosalpingography.
Based on data of Henry-Suchet *et al.* (1984).

4.2 HYSTEROSALPINGOGRAPHY

Hysterosalpingography is the most common and some-times the only fertility investigation to be undertaken, and provides accurate morphological information, especially regarding the uterine cavity and proximal fallopian tube. Hysterosalpingography is best per-formed towards the end of the first week after the menstrual period when the isthmus is most distensible and the fallopian tubes are most readily filled by con-trast medium. It should only be performed in the second half of the menstrual cycle if adequate contraception has been used, or if there is evidence that pregnancy is unlikely.

Some authors, including Palmer (1960) and De-Cherny et al. (1980), ascribe a therapeutic effect to hysterosalpingography. Others (Cumming & Taylor, 1979), however, have advocated the combined use of hysteroscopy and laparoscopy for evaluating the uterus and fallopian tubes, to the exclusion of hysterosalpingo-graphy. Nevertheless, hysterosalpingography is gene-rally the first investigation to be performed as it is considered to be less invasive than endoscopy. In low risk patients it provides a safe and reasonably produc-tive method of investigating the genital tract.

Technique

Hysterosalpingography is performed in the radiology department, usually without anaesthesia, using fluoro-scopy and image intensification and with the facility to take multiple films during the procedure. Diazepam can be given orally before the examination, but mor-phine and pethidine should not be used as they can cause the smooth muscle of the tubes to contract. The patient lies in the dorsal position with her legs flexed during insertion of a cervical cannula; her legs are then straightened with the feet slightly apart for the examination.

Most radiologists use a water-soluble medium which should be sufficiently dense to give adequate contrast and yet viscid enough not to leak into the vagina or flow through the tubes too quickly. Water-soluble media disappear within one hour from the peritoneal cavity and within a few hours from hydro-salpinges.

A preliminary plain film is necessary not only to identify pelvic opacities but also to act as a guide to the correct exposure. 5–10 ml of contrast medium is then injected slowly while screening so that the uterine cavity and tubes can be examined, and filling defects can be seen before they are obscured by the medium. If there is bilateral proximal tubal obstruction, there is resist-ance to the plunger of the syringe and the patient experiences mild lower abdominal pain due to uterine

distension. If one tube is freely patent, passage of dye along the contralateral tube may be delayed, giving a false impression of proximal obstruction. If this occurs, a further 1–4 ml of contrast medium should be injected and time should be allowed for the tubal orifice to relax and open. Occasionally there may be genuine tubal spasm in which case a relaxant drug such as amylnitrite can be used, although it causes unpleasant side-effects. If the patient is under general anaesthesia, halothane causes relaxation of the muscle. Glucagon given intravenously in doses of 2 ml can also be used to reverse spasm of the intramural segment of the tube.

Normal Findings

Normally, as the uterus fills with contrast medium, the cornua are seen to be spindle shaped, and the apex of the cornu is seen to be continuous with the lumen of the intramural segment of the tube. There may be a pretubal bulge caused by an anatomical fold separating the endometrium from the endosalpinx.

The intramural portion of the tube can usually be visualized and, if there is proximal obstruction, the exact site of the blockage can be identified (Fig. 4.2.1). The luminal wall of the intramural tube and isthmus should be smooth and of uniform diameter. When the dye flows into the ampulla, the mucosal folds are clear-ly seen before the tube is completely filled (Fig. 4.2.2). The ampulla is 5–6 cm long with a varying degree of tortuosity. When the contrast medium spills from the fimbrial end of the tube it becomes dispersed between loops of bowel.

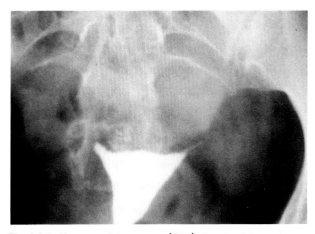

Fig. 4.2.1 Hysterosalpingogram (HSG) showing bilateral blockage of the intramural segment of the fallopian tubes.

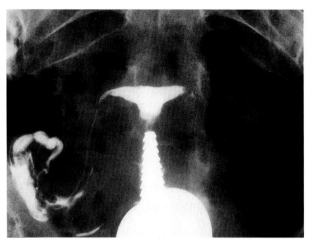

Fig. 4.2.2 HSG showing normal mucosal folds in the ampulla of the right tube.
Left salpingectomy has previously been performed for a ruptured tubal pregnancy.

Abnormal Findings

A number of acquired conditions may be diagnosed by hysterosalpingography. In some, for example distal tubal obstruction, there may be difficulty in interpreting the findings, but in others, such as salpingitis isthmica nodosa, the radiological appearance is typical and is the most accurate method of making the diagnosis.

Distal Tubal Obstruction
In distal tubal obstruction there is no spillage of contrast medium and a varying degree of ampullary dilatation (Figs 4.2.3 & 4.2.4). Often the obstruction is incomplete or there are peritubal adhesions causing the dye to become loculated in which case there may be no dilatation of the ampulla. Loculation is confirmed by noting that the appearance of the dye does not change with the position of the patient. Peritubal adhesions may fix the tubes in an abnormal position when there may be convolution of both ampulla and isthmus.

Salpingitis Isthmica Nodosa
Salpingitis isthmica nodosa is characterized by diverticula of varying size, usually about 2 mm in diameter, arising from a segment of the isthmus, 1–2 cm long, of one or both tubes (Fig. 4.2.5). The continuity of the smooth tubal lumen is interrupted and flecks of contrast material appear at a short distance above or below the lumen. Salpingitis isthmica nodosa is bilateral in almost 50% of cases.

Tubal Endometriosis
In tubal endometriosis, the isthmus has a honeycomb appearance but remains patent. There are diverticula which are thicker than in salpingitis isthmica nodosa

although it is possible that one is merely a variant of the other.

Tuberculosis
Tuberculosis of the genital tract is still a major cause of infertility in many countries. It may mimic the radiological appearance of salpingitis isthmica nodosa, but the nodules are less uniform and the tube is more rigid with small terminal sacculations. There may be calcification in the tubes, ovaries and pelvic lymph nodes. The tubes are frequently blocked on both sides, and are usually moderately dilated with a club-shaped appearance of the ampulla (Fig. 4.2.6). Tuberculosis is suggested on hysterosalpingography by gross thickening of the longitudinal mucosal folds, but the contour may be smooth or irregular, and there may be cavities or even multiple strictures, which give the tube a beaded appearance. Small sinuses may also be seen, and the tube may have a rigid or 'pipe stem' appearance, or be fixed in an abnormal position by adhesions. Rarely tubointestinal fistulae may occur.

Tubal Polyps
Tubal polyps are seen as oval shadows in the intramural segment with contrast medium flowing in a thin line above or below them. David *et al.* (1981), reported the presence of bilateral polyps in 2.5% of hysterosalpingograms, but disputed their relationship to infertility.

Ovarian Cysts
The tube may be stretched over a large ovarian cyst so that it appears distorted and partially obstructed. The cyst wall may be outlined by dye which has spilled into the peritoneal cavity.

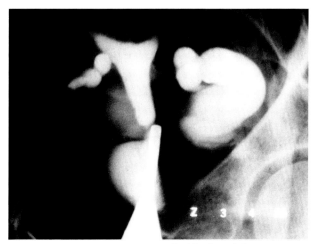

Fig. 4.2.3 HSG showing a thin-walled hydrosalpinx.
There is marked distension of the ampulla but no spillage of contrast medium into the peritoneal cavity.

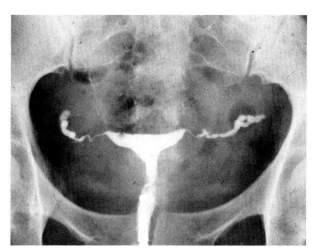

Fig. 4.2.4 HSG showing a thick-walled hydrosalpinx.
There is distal tubal blockage, but little dilatation of the ampulla due to the thick walls.

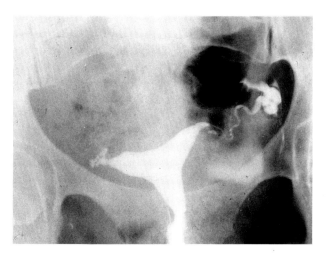

Fig. 4.2.5 Salpingitis isthmica nodosa.
HSG showing the typical small nodules along the isthmic segment of both tubes.

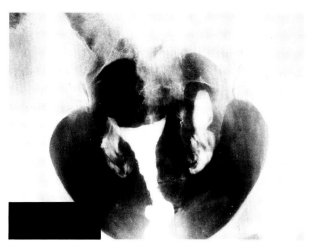

Fig. 4.2.6 Tuberculous salpingitis.
This shows bilateral distal tubal obstruction and the club-shaped appearance of the ampulla.

Pelvic Endometriosis
Extensive pelvic endometriosis causes fixation of the uterus, usually in retroflexion, and dilatation of the ampulla due to adhesions may be seen. It is impossible to distinguish endometriosis from pelvic inflammatory disease by hysterosalpingography alone.

Congenital and Acquired Anomalies
Few congenital anomalies of the tube can be demonstrated by hysterosalpingography. On the other hand, acquired abnormalities of the isthmus and intramural segment, which are more common, can only be diagnosed with certainty by this technique, although there may be confirmatory signs on endoscopy.

Complications

Although hysterosalpingography is an outpatient procedure which can be performed with little discomfort to the patient and without analgesia, it is not without complication. The use of water-soluble media has eliminated the risk of oil embolism and granuloma formation, and fluoroscopy and image intensification has reduced the incidence of intravasation of medium.

Infection
Infection remains a hazard and its sequelae may cause infertility resulting from tubal damage. The incidence of infection following the injection of radio-opaque

dye has been variously reported, as 0.3% (Marshak, 1950), 1.3% (Measday, 1960) and 3.1% (Stumph & March, 1980). The latter study was prospective and a number of those women who developed infection were seriously ill following the procedure; prophylactic antibiotics did not appear to reduce the risk and those who developed pelvic infection could not be identified by any preoperative laboratory investigation.

Most of the women who develop pelvic infection following hysterosalpingography have distal tubal disease and it is rare for women with normal tubes or proximal disease to develop pelvic peritonitis.

Irradiation of an Early Embryo

Irradiation of an early embryo is possible if the investigation is performed during the luteal phase, though the risk to the embryo is small. Nevertheless the '10 day rule' should be observed.

Pain

Pain during the examination is usually transient and mild and can be minimized by injecting the contrast medium slowly, using no more than is necessary. Application of a tenaculum can cause bleeding from the cervix; this can be avoided by using a different type of cannula.

Allergy

The patient should be questioned about allergies; if there is doubt, laparoscopy should be performed instead of hysterosalpingography.

Radionuclide Hysterosalpingography

Although it is recognized that some anatomically normal tubes have defective cilial function and, conversely, that the transport mechanism may be normal in tubes with partial or complete obstruction, there is no established clinical method for investigating the function of the fallopian tube in the human. The recognition of such functional disorders is important for the correct selection of patients for tubal surgery, *in vitro* fertilization and gamete intrafallopian transfer. Studies of sperm transport to the pouch of Douglas by a combined post-coital test and laparoscopy have not gained general acceptance in clinical practice and there are logistic problems in both the performance and timing of the procedure. However, Brundin *et al.* (1989), have recently described a method of evaluating the capacity of the tubal epithelium to transport particles using radionuclide hysterosalpingography (RN-HSG).

In 1981, Iturralde and Venter described the spontaneous migration of inert technetium-labelled human albumin microspheres from the vagina to the fallopian tubes and ovaries, and suggested that this method of transport could convey carcinogens to the ovaries. McCalley *et al.* (1985), later described a similar test to confirm tubal patency in the investigation of infertility. They suggested that although sperm motility was essential for penetration of the ovum, it may not be the basic factor in sperm transport.

Subsequently, Brundin *et al.* (1989), have investigated infertile women using standard HSG and RN-HSG to compare the morphological appearance of the fallopian tube with its ability to transport particulate matter. HSG was carried out using sufficient contrast medium to fill both tubes when they were intact. Approximately 1–4 months later RN-HSG was performed 1–2 days before ovulation as estimated by basal body temperature charts during the two preceding months. The patients were asked to abstain from intercourse for one week prior to the test. Technetium-labelled microspheres of human albumin with a diameter of 10–20 μg were slowly instilled into the cervix on day 11–13 of the cycle and any fluid which leaked back into the vagina was measured with an isotope calibrator. It was considered important not to inject the microspheres under pressure as their deposition in the uterine cavity would invalidate the results. Transport of the microspheres was measured by serial gamma camera examinations over the following 8 hours.

Fig. 4.2.7a shows a normal HSG with bilateral tubal patency, but Fig. 4.2.7b shows that the microspheres were transported to the ovary on the left side whereas on the right side they only reached the intramural segment of the tube. This suggests a defect in tubal function on the right side despite normal anatomy. The HSG shown in Fig. 4.2.8a shows a left-sided hydrosalpinx and failure of filling of the right tube, but the RN-HSG (Fig. 4.2.8b) shows passage of the microspheres into both tubal ampullae suggesting that the transport mechanism is intact and that normal function might be restored by tubal reconstructive surgery.

In Brundin's series, 26 tubes were considered normal and patent on HSG, but there was no transport of the microspheres on RN-HSG in 14 of them, suggesting a defect in tubal function despite normal morphology. Nine tubes had distal blockage with hydrosalpinx formation, but in four of these the microspheres were transported normally towards the distal tube suggesting that the transport mechanism was intact (Fig. 4.2.9). After 18 months' follow-up, two patients whose HSG and RN-HSG were both normal had conceived, whereas none of the women with a normal HSG but an abnormal RN-HSG had become pregnant.

Further work is required, but the initial impression is that RN-HSG could be used in combination with other tests of tubal morphology to detect a possible cause of unexplained infertility when the tubes are patent and apparently normal.

RN-HSG could also be of value in deciding whether to offer tubal reconstructive surgery or *in vitro* fertilization to women with distal tubal obstruction, and in recognizing the woman with apparently normal tubes in whom gamete intrafallopian transfer might be contra-indicated because of a defective transport mechanism.

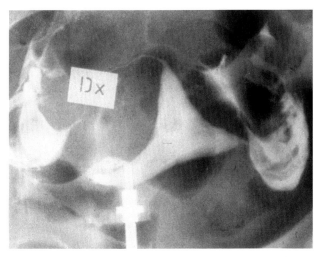

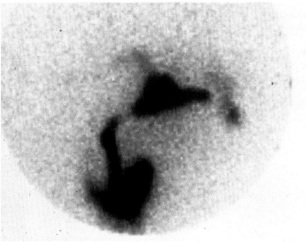

Fig. 4.2.7a & b Patent tubes with defective function.
a HSG shows normal fallopian tubes with bilateral patency.

b RN-HSG shows transport of microspheres to the left fimbriae and ovary, but only to the intramural segment of the right tube.

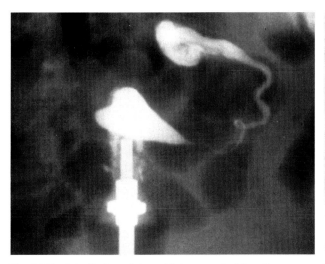

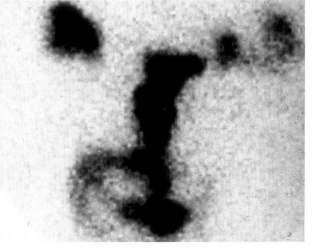

Fig. 4.2.8a & b Hydrosalpinx with intact tubal function.
a HSG shows distal obstruction on the left side and no filling of the right tube.

b RN-HSG shows transport of the microspheres to the ampulla of both tubes and confirms bilateral hydrosalpinx.

		HSG	
		Tube patent	Tube obstructed
RN-HSG	Tube patent	12	4
	Tube obstructed	14	5

Fig. 4.2.9 Hysterosalpingography (HSG) vs radionuclide hysterosalpingography (RN-HSG) in the assessment of tubal function.

4.3 HYSTEROSCOPY

B.J. van Herendael, M. Stevens, T. Slangen and A.M. Van Bel

Hysteroscopy may be performed as an office procedure, but is probably better combined with other endoscopic investigations. The complication rate is low, and the popularity of this procedure has increased in the last 18 years since the introduction of carbon dioxide gas insufflation by Lindemann in 1971.

Hysteroscopy enables inspection of the uterine cavity in detail and also visualization of the internal ostium and the proximal intramural segment of the fallopian tube. Hysterosalpingography and hysteroscopy correlate well in the diagnosis of malformations of the Mullerian duct, but in the assessment of synechiae, submucous fibroids and polyps their correlation is poor.

Examination of the tubal ostium by hysteroscopy demonstrates the normal activity of the peri-orificial musculature and failure to appreciate this may lead to an incorrect diagnosis of proximal tubal obstruction. However, hysteroscopy is a poor indicator of tubal patency, and the integrity of the intramural and isthmic segments of the tube need to be assessed by hysterosalpingography and laparoscopy.

Technique

In order to perform hysteroscopy, the uterine cavity needs to be inflated. This is achieved by an automatic insufflator delivering carbon dioxide at a preselected rate whilst also maintaining an intra-uterine pressure of 50–80 mm Hg, but not exceeding 100 mm Hg. Alternatively, various fluid media can be used instead of carbon dioxide, such as the high molecular weight fluids, Hyskon or Dextran, which are preferable to saline or dextrose solution. Hyskon should be used in operative procedures where bleeding may occur as it is immiscible with blood and the fluid medium remains clear.

In investigative work the normal panhysteroscope with a 30 degree oblique angle is used, but for a more detailed examination of the endometrium and tubal ostia the contact microcolpohysteroscope (Hamou, 1980), which magnifies up to ×60 is required. After careful introduction into the insufflated uterine cavity, the hysteroscope is advanced to within 2 cm of the fundus, when rotation of the telescope on its axis

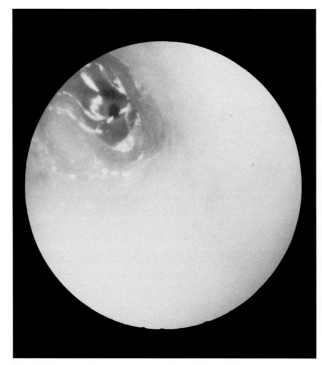

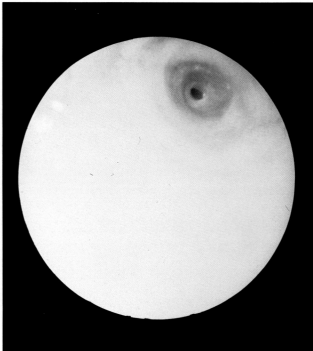

Fig. 4.3.1a & b Hysteroscopic view of the ostium.
a The right tubal ostium with reflections from a gas bubble.

b After the gas bubble passes through, the tubal ostium remains open for a while.

through 90 degrees will bring the tubal ostium into view. The telescope is then moved towards the ostium. The lens system produces ×20 magnification when the optic is 1 cm from the surface; this magnification permits a detailed study of the endometrium and tubal orifice. When the telescope is in contact with the surface the magnification can be increased to ×60 so that the endometrial vascular pattern can be examined.

Normal Findings

During observation of the tubal orifice, the insufflating gas can be seen to flow out through the ostium when the intrauterine pressure exceeds that in the fallopian tube. The tubal orifice, which is initially closed, slowly opens as the intrauterine pressure is increased, enabling visualization of the interior of the proximal intramural segment. The ostium remains dilated whilst the gas passes through and then gradually closes. An air bubble is shown collecting in the uterine cornu before slipping into the tube, which then remains open for a while

(Fig. 4.3.1). In this way the tubal ostium can be studied and the changes in its appearance in different phases of the menstrual cycle can be observed. It must be remembered, however, that the uterus is artificially distended in hysteroscopy and not in its normal physiological state, so observations on the activity of the uterine and tubal muscle should be interpreted with this in mind.

The appearance of the endometrium and epithelium of the intramural portion of the tube varies in the different phases of the menstrual cycle and normally there is a clear delineation between the two. During the proliferative phase, the epithelium of the intramural tube is vascular and appears redder than the surrounding endometrium. There is a crescentic membrane (Fig. 4.3.2a) at the boundary, but the actual ostium is round and central in the uterine cornu. During the secretory phase, on the other hand, the tubal epithelium becomes paler and thicker, the ostium is less well defined and the membrane often becomes transparent (Fig. 4.3.2b), so the differentiation between the two membranes is not so distinct.

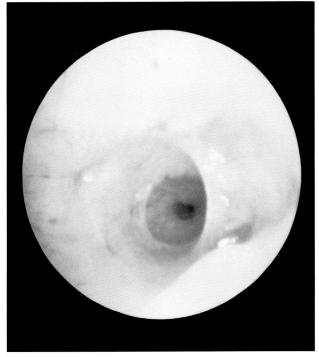

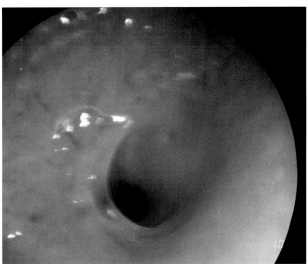

Fig. 4.3.2a & b The crescentic membrane.
a At hysteroscopy, the crescentic membrane is seen at the boundary between the endometrium and endosalpinx. The tubal ostium is open.

b During the secretory phase, the crescentic membrane is transparent.

Abnormal Findings

Pathological conditions produce characteristic changes in the hysteroscopic view of the endometrium and fallopian tube.

Acute Endometritis

Acute endometritis involving the whole uterine cavity (Fig. 4.3.3a) causes changes in both the tubal ostium and the intramural portion of the tube. There is vascular hyperaemia (Fig. 4.3.3b) with local bleeding, and the border between the tube and endometrium becomes less distinct than usual. The tubal epithelium also undergoes a hyperplastic reaction giving it an irregular outline.

Partial Obstruction of the Ostium

Partial obstruction of the ostium is caused by tubo-cornual myomata and polyps. Fig. 4.3.4 shows several polyps protruding from the tubal opening but these are probably reactionary and evidence of pathology in the tube rather than primary lesions in the meatus.

Fibrosis

Occasionally an infectious process in the tube leads to fibrosis in the ostium which becomes irregular in shape with hard, white, avascular tissue surrounding it (Fig. 4.3.5). The degree of fibrosis varies from mild, with some white areas in the endometrium, to severe, with dense fibrous tissue which obliterates the whole ostium.

Acute Salpingitis

Acute salpingitis affecting the medial segments of the tube leads to the formation of new blood vessels in the mucosa with numerous connecting branches, which spread from the tubal ostium radially over the endometrium (Fig. 4.3.6a). The ostium is rounded but its edges are indistinct due to hyperplasia of the intramural mucosa. Occasionally the ostium shrinks and appears as a red dot (Fig. 4.3.6b).

Salpingitis Isthmica Nodosa

Salpingitis isthmica nodosa produces a typical appearance in the intramural mucosa, which is hyperplastic

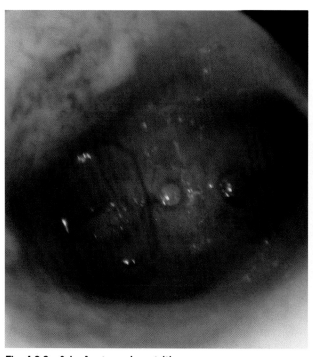

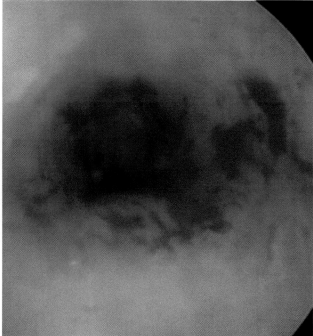

Fig. 4.3.3a & b Acute endometritis.
a A panoramic view of the uterine cavity showing the increased vascularity of the endometrium with small haemorrhages.

b Close up view of the uterine cornu.

with enlarged tubal folds, possibly due to focal hormonal influences. Also the normally round ostium is irregular in outline and less well-defined due to the enlarged folds, and the border between the tubal mucosa and endometrium is poorly delineated (Fig. 4.3.7).

Extra-uterine Pregnancy

Extra-uterine pregnancy is characterized by a dilated tubal orifice and blood can be seen to trickle through the ostium into the uterine cavity when the pregnancy begins to abort (Fig. 4.3.8).

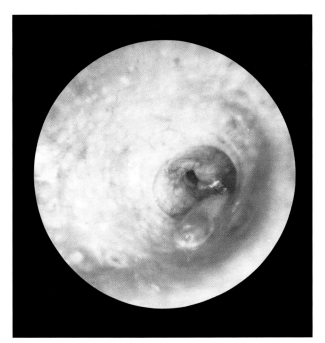

Fig. 4.3.4 Tubocornual polyps.

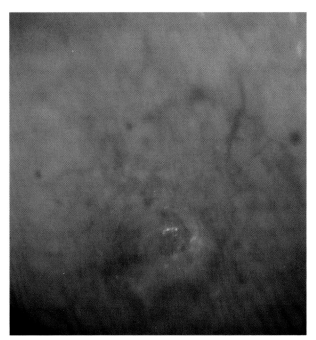

Fig. 4.3.5 Fibrosis.
Chronic salpingitis results in dense fibrous tissue formation around the tubal ostium.

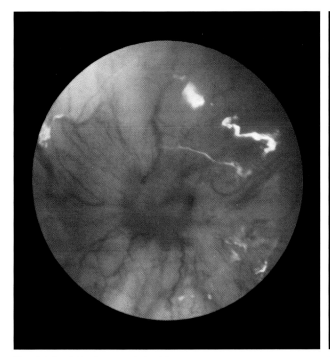

Fig. 4.3.6a & b Acute salpingitis.
a Note the radial spread of new blood vessels.

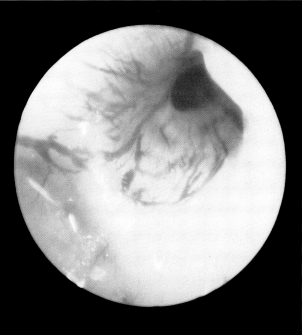

b The ostium is small and appears as a red dot.

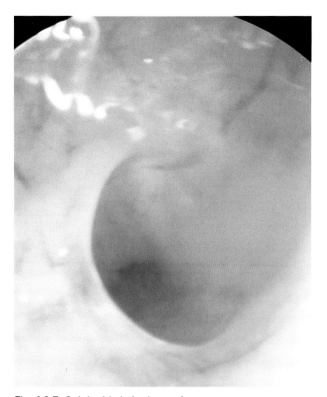

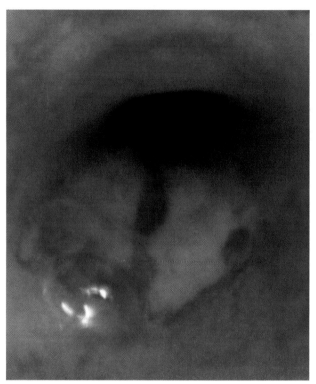

Fig. 4.3.7 Salpingitis isthmica nodosa.
The prominent mucosal folds in the intramural segment can be
clearly seen.

Fig. 4.3.8 Aborting ectopic pregnancy.
Blood can be seen trickling through the ostium.

4.4 LAPAROSCOPY

Laparoscopy is a well-established technique in the
routine investigation and treatment of infertility. It
allows a complete and detailed examination of the pelvic
organs and the pelvic and abdominal peritoneum, and a
superficial examination of the bowel, liver and inferior
surface of the diaphragm.

Complications can occur even with experienced
operators, although the risk is directly proportional to
the skill of the surgeon. In the British Laparoscopy
Survey (Chamberlain & Carron Brown, 1977), there
were four deaths resulting from 50,247 operations and
the complication rate was greater for those regions
where fewer laparoscopies were performed. Phillips *et
al.* (1975), stressed that it takes 250 laparoscopies to
develop the skill to be a safe operator, and that the
learning period must be supervised by an experienced
laparoscopist.

Technique

Laparoscopy must always be performed in a fully
equipped operating theatre so that any complication
which might arise can be treated without moving the
patient to another theatre or hospital. Appropriate
instruments for performing operative laparoscopy
should be immediately available and it must always be
possible to proceed to laparotomy without delay if
complications develop.

Full examination of an infertile patient by hysteroscopy, laparoscopy and salpingoscopy may take 45–90
minutes. The patient should therefore be anaesthetized
using muscle relaxants, endotracheal intubation and
positive pressure respiration. The patient's blood pressure and heart rate must be monitored continuously
throughout the operation.

Closed circuit television is a great advantage, not
only for teaching purposes, but also to allow the
surgeon to operate in a more comfortable position
either with conventional instruments or laser, by view-
ing the video screen instead of operating through the
lens.

Routine laparoscopy is performed using either an
operating laparoscope with a probe passed down the
operating channel, or a standard laparoscope with a
probe or forceps introduced through a second incision.
After panoramic inspection of the pelvis with the uterus
in its normal position, the uterus is retroverted to
allow inspection of the uterovesical pouch before
examination of the fundus and cornua in detail.

Uterus

The general appearance of the uterus is observed while any factors which could influence fertility, such as intramural or subserous fibroids, or defects in fusion of the Mullerian ducts are looked for. In these latter cases the relationship of the round ligament, fallopian tube and ovarian ligament should be noted and the correct anatomy defined.

The Fallopian Tubes

Following inspection of the uterus, the fallopian tubes are examined in detail. They must be visualized throughout their length from cornua to fimbriae with the lens close to the objective so that any peritoneal defects or adhesions can be clearly seen. Proximal blockage will be evident if dye fails to fill the tubal lumen, and if pressure on the syringe causes the dye to intravasate giving a blue coloration to the uterine fundus (Fig. 4.4.1). Irregularities in the isthmus may indicate endometriosis or salpingitis isthmica nodosa (Fig. 4.4.2), which can be confirmed when chromopertubation is performed. The diverticula of salpingitis isthmica nodosa can be identified when they fill with dye and small blue spots are seen beneath the tubal serosa.

During examination of the ampulla its diameter and mobility should be noted, while adhesions between the tube and ovary which limit peristaltic movement (Fig. 4.4.3) and surface lesions, such as endometriotic spots, should be looked for (Fig. 4.4.4). The fimbriae are then

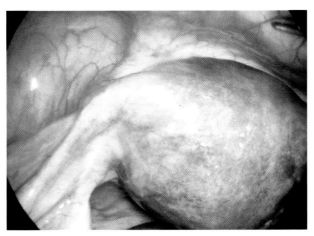

Fig. 4.4.1 Proximal blockage of the fallopian tube.
Intravasation of methylene blue suggests proximal tubal obstruction. (Courtesy of Dr Alain Audebert.)

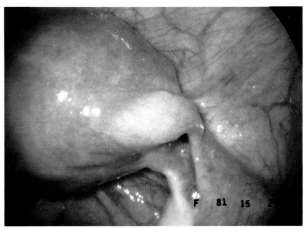

Fig. 4.4.2 Irregularity of the isthmus.
Swelling of the proximal isthmus suggests endometriosis or salpingitis isthmica nodosa.

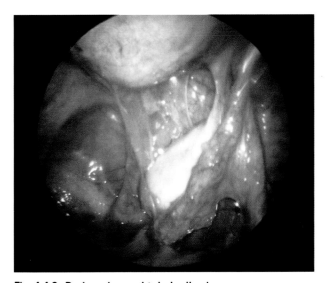

Fig. 4.4.3 Periovarian and tubal adhesions.
Adhesions interfere with ovum pick-up and limit tubal mobility.

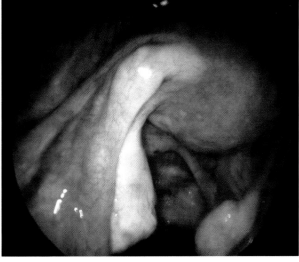

Fig. 4.4.4 Isthmic endometriosis.
There is also a chronic tubal pregnancy.

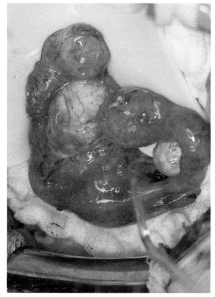
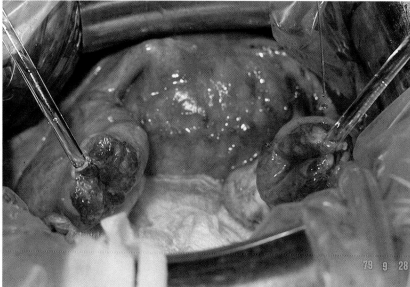

Fig. 4.4.5a & b Thin-walled hydrosalpinx.
a A thin-walled hydrosalpinx characterized by a transparent, irregularly distended tube.

b Thin-walled hydrosalpinx after salpingostomy.

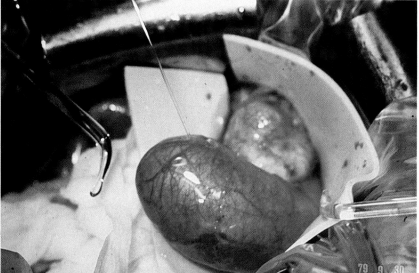
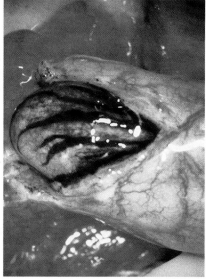

Fig. 4.4.6a & b Thick-walled hydrosalpinx.
a A thick-walled hydrosalpinx characterized by a regular distension of the tube, which unlike that of a thin-walled hydrosalpinx, is opaque.

b Salpingostomy demonstrates the thickened tubal wall.

closely inspected for evidence of fimbrial adhesions which might indicate mucosal damage, and finally, the normality of the fimbria ovarica must be confirmed. If there is distal blockage, the dilated ampulla must be examined in detail to determine whether the hydrosalpinx is thin or thick walled (Figs 4.4.5 & 4.4.6) and to identify the presence of the star at the point of the blockage (Fig. 4.4.7).

Incidental Infection or Unsuspected Tubal Pregnancy
An acute condition such as infection or unsuspected tubal pregnancy may be encountered during the endoscopic investigation of infertility. If acute infection is diagnosed, repeat laparoscopy and salpingoscopy should be considered following treatment to detect tubal mucosal damage. The diagnosis of chronic infection caused by *Chlamydia trachomatis* or

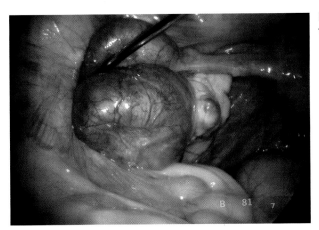

Fig. 4.4.7 Thin-walled hydrosalpinx.
The star-shaped scar is clearly seen at the point of blockage.

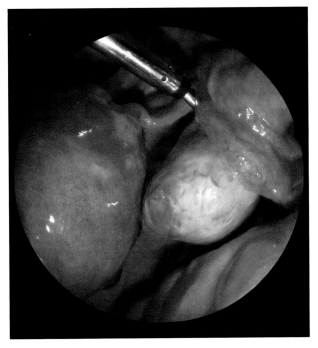

Fig. 4.4.8 Ovulation.
The stigma at the site of ovulation is seen on the medial aspect
of the ovary.

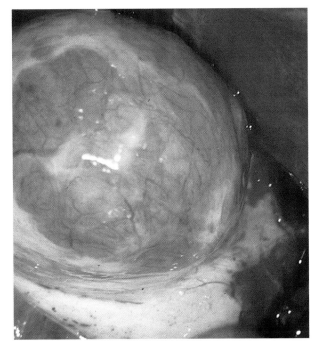

Fig. 4.4.9 Luteinization of unruptured follicle.
There is no stigma.

Mycobacterium tuberculosis needs to be confirmed by culture of intratubal or peritoneal fluid.

A tubal mole can be left without treatment if the titre of human chorionic gonatrophin (HCG) is falling. Alternatively cytotoxic drugs may be given. When an unruptured tubal pregnancy is discovered, salpingoscopy should first be performed to determine the state of the mucosa in both tubes before deciding whether or not to carry out conservative tubal surgery. If the mucosa is healthy and the tubal anatomy has not been disrupted by the pregnancy, conservative surgery can be performed using laparoscopic or microsurgical techniques. However, if the tube is disrupted or if there is evidence of mucosal damage resulting from a previous infection, laparoscopic salpingectomy is the correct treatment if the pregnancy is in the ampulla, whereas if it is in the cornu or medial isthmus, laparotomy and removal of the tube will be necessary.

Small fimbrial cysts can be left *in situ* but larger ones which may interfere with tubal mobility should be removed.

Ovaries

The ovaries are inspected carefully noting any evidence of ovarian activity; follicular and luteal cysts and the stigma at the site of ovulation are looked for (Fig. 4.4.8). Evidence of ovulatory disorders are frequently found during infertility investigations(Fig. 4.4.9). The enlarged ovary of polycystic ovarian disease is easily recognized. Although the diagnosis can be confirmed

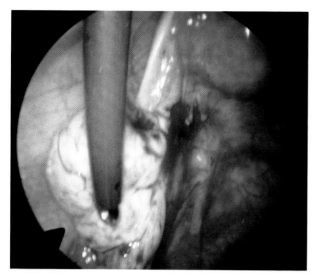

Fig. 4.4.10 Ovarian endometriosis.
Adhesions between the ovary and the broad ligament have been divided, thereby mobilizing the ovary.

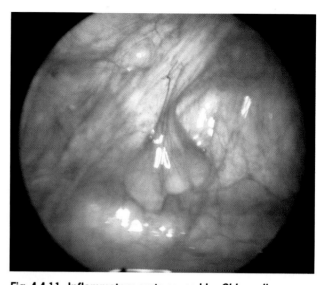

Fig. 4.4.11 Inflammatory cysts caused by *Chlamydia trachomatis*.
Inflammatory cysts can be seen on the left utero-sacral ligament.

by biopsy, it is more commonly diagnosed by a combination of ultrasound and an elevated ratio of luteinizing hormone (LH) to follicle stimulating hormone (FSH). The hypotrophic ovaries of anorexia nervosa and Turner's syndrome are similarly small and without signs of activity.

The surface of the ovaries is examined for endometriosis, or adhesions between the tube and ovary or between the ovary and broad ligament (Fig. 4.4.10). The ovaries are then lifted with forceps to expose their lateral aspect and, again, signs of endometriosis or adhesions are looked for. Inflammatory cysts, which are common in *Chlamydia trachomatis* infection, are usually situated on the posterior surface of the uterus or on the ovaries (Fig. 4.4.11).

Pelvic Peritoneum

Examination of the pelvic peritoneum should proceed in a clockwise direction commencing with the anterior abdominal wall, then moving to the right utero-vesical fold, the anterior surface of the right broad ligament, the round ligament, the fallopian tube, the posterior surface of the broad ligament and the pouch of Douglas

and back to the utero-vesical pouch via the left side. Any adhesions between the ovaries, large or small bowel, uterus, broad ligament or the floor of the pouch should be noted.

It may be difficult to differentiate between adhesions caused by pelvic inflammatory disease and those resulting from endometriosis. This differentiation can usually be made, however, by salpingoscopy, as pelvic inflammatory disease is often associated with adhesions between the mucosal folds of the fallopian tube whereas endometriosis does not produce intratubal lesions.

Endometriosis

During laparoscopy, hormonally-active endometriosis of the peritoneum appears as small, fresh papules on the peritoneal surface of the broad ligament and on the floor of the pouch of Douglas (Fig.4.4.12a). The papules are 1–2 mm in diameter and look like tiny blisters in the peritoneum. On histological examination these papules are found to consist of typical healthy endometrium with a normal vascular pattern consistent with the phase of the menstrual cycle. They should not be confused with other white papules containing foreign bodies or representing hyperplastic mesothelium, which

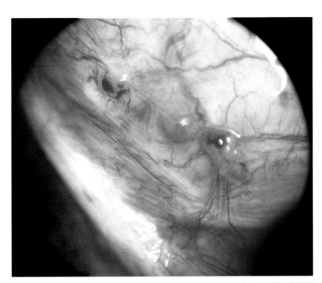

Fig. 4.4.12a–c Peritoneal endometriosis.
a Clear blisters can be seen on the posterior surface of the broad ligament indicating hormonally-active endometriosis.

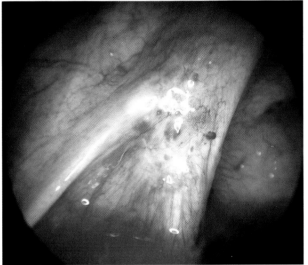

b 'Powder-burn' lesions on the left utero-sacral ligament.

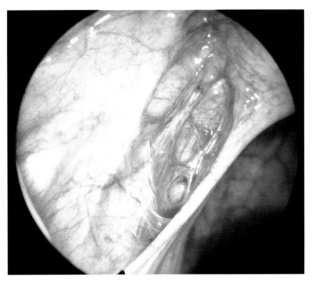

c Peritoneal defect caused by contraction of fibrous tissue resulting from endometriosis.

are common on the tubal peritoneum and have no clinical significance. In peritoneal endometriosis there is also an increase in the number of fine vessels in the peritoneum around the vesicle and, sometimes, this vascular change is the only visible sign of this condition. Again, biopsy of the peritoneum will confirm the diagnosis.

The diagnosis of endometriosis of the pelvic peritoneum is most commonly based on finding haemorrhagic or black foci with fibrosis, forming the classic 'powder-burn' lesions (Fig. 4.4.12b). Contraction of the fibrous tissue together with retraction of the surface peritoneum leads to peritoneal defects (Fig. 4.4.12c) which, when examined closely, have foci of endometriosis at their bases. The sequelae of endometriosis, which include adhesions with fibrosis, pseudo-peritoneal cysts and endometriomata may not represent active disease. Although these lesions may require surgery to alleviate pain, this will have little effect on fertility. Alternatively, suppressive treatment with danazol or gonadotrophic releasing hormone agonists may be helpful.

The Abdominal Cavity

Following inspection of the pelvic organs the abdominal cavity is then examined systematically. The appendix is identified and its visual normality confirmed as previous appendicular disease is a common cause of tubal disease, especially on the right side. The descending and sigmoid colon are inspected for evidence of diverticular disease and its consistency is determined by palpation with a probe. The paracolic gutters which frequently contain endometriosis, are inspected for evidence of disease or adhesions. Finally the liver and inferior surface of the diaphragm are examined for adhesions which may indicate gonococcal or chlamydial infection (Fig. 4.4.13).

Operative Laparoscopy

The modern laparoscopist should be able to proceed from diagnostic to operative laparoscopy using either coagulation and scissor dissection or laser to divide adhesions resulting from pelvic inflammatory disease and to treat endometriosis (see page 5.20). This obviates the need for laparotomy in a significant number of

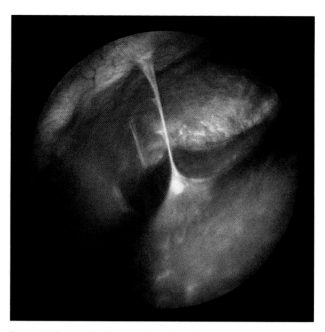

Fig. 4.4.13 Subdiaphragmatic adhesion.

cases and often gives better results. The limitations of laparoscopic surgery should, however, be recognized and the place of tubal microsurgery remembered.

4.5   SALPINGOSCOPY

Until recently there has been no endoscopic means of examining the tubal mucosa and it had to be assumed that tubal patency equated with tubal normality. Laparoscopic salpingoscopy permits detailed examination of the endosalpinx as an adjunct to other investigations of tubal function. It is a logical extension of the endoscopic examination of the female genital tract.

Indications

The indications for salpingoscopy are as follows.
1. Unsuspected tubal mucosal lesions may be revealed, a significant number of which are not detected during hysterosalpingography. These include adhesions, flattening of the mucosal folds or complete loss of the normal fold pattern, all of which can occur even when the tubes are patent.
2. The extent of mucosal damage in the woman who has had pelvic inflammatory disease can be assessed so that she can be counselled regarding her future fertility.
3. The status of the tubal mucosa in patients who have established tubal disease with adhesions or hydrosalpinx can be assessed. This can avoid unnecessary laparotomy, as microsurgery is unlikely to be successful if the mucosa is damaged. Boer-Meisel *et al.* (1986), used the operating microscope to examine the distal segment of

the fallopian tube and found that a pregnancy rate of 77% could be achieved following salpingostomy for thin-walled hydrosalpinx if the mucosa was normal. In the case of distal blockage, the hydrosalpinx must be opened before introducing the telescope. In cases of proximal blockage where tubo-cornual anastomosis is under consideration, it is essential that the ampullary mucosa is inspected first because there may also be ampullary mucosal damage which would make surgery unsuccessful.
4. In ectopic pregnancy, if the tubal mucosa is damaged in the affected or the contralateral side, preservation of that tube will not improve the patient's fertility and may lead to a further ectopic implantation.
5. Prior to gamete intrafallopian transfer (GIFT), mucosal lesions which could interfere with transport of the gametes can be excluded and difficulties in cannulating the tubal ostium can be identified.

Instruments

For many years gynaecologists have been examining the tubal mucosa of infertile patients during tubal reconstructive surgery. Mohri *et al.* (1970), described a hysteroscopic method using a glassfibre telescope, but the value of the procedure was limited by the quality of the optical system. More recently laparoscopic techniques have been developed which use a variety of telescopes to gain access to the tubal lumen. These have included modified hysteroscopes inserted through a separate incision, and flexible bronchoscopes (Cornier, 1982 & 1985) introduced through an operating laparoscope. Currently a series of specially designed rigid salpingoscopes have been developed to allow salpingoscopy to become a standard endoscopic procedure in the investigation of infertility (Brosens *et al.*, 1987).

Endoscopic examination of the tubal mucosa can be performed during diagnostic laparoscopy using a salpingoscope introduced through the channel of an operating laparoscope.

The component parts of the salpingoscope are shown in Fig. 4.5.1 and consist of the operating laparoscope, the sheath of the salpingoscope which is 5 mm in diameter and has a connector for a saline infusion, an obturator with its rounded end to aid introduction, and a 3 mm telescope.

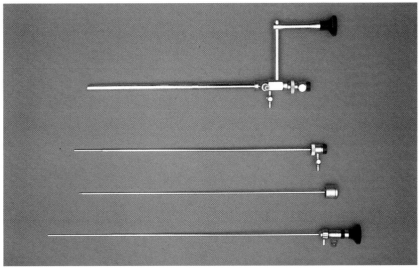

Fig. 4.5.1a–d Instruments for salpingoscopy.
a From above, the operating laparoscope, the sheath, the obturator and the salpingoscope.

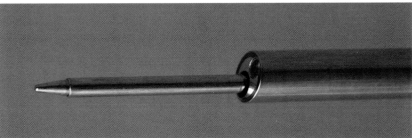

b The sheath with the obturator protruding from the laparoscope.

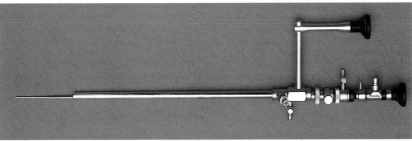

c The assembled salpingoscope.

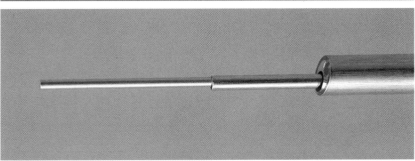

d The salpingoscope protruding from the sheath.

Technique

The patient should be prepared for routine laparoscopy (see page 4.12), the bladder emptied, and an intrauterine cannula inserted and attached to the cervix to facilitate manipulation of the uterus. Laparoscopy with the normal detailed examination of the pelvic cavity can then be performed. The uterus is then anteverted and the adnexa lifted forwards with tube-holding forceps before retroverting and rotating it through 90 degrees. Following this the uterus is displaced laterally so that the fundus lies in the ovarian fossa with the tube and ovary on its anterior surface. The tube can then be gently manipulated with the forceps to align it with the laparoscope (Fig. 4.5.2).

The sheath with its obturator is then passed down the operating channel. The fimbrial opening, which is near the antimesenteric border of the tube is identified and the laparoscope is brought close to the tube to allow the sheath to advance slowly out of the operating channel and into the tubal infundibulum. If necessary, the fimbriae can be steadied by grasping them with tube-holding forceps which must be repositioned once the sheath is in the tube to grasp its full circumference and form a water-tight seal. The obturator is removed and replaced by the telescope.

A saline infusion is now commenced and the tube is seen to distend. This is an essential part of the procedure which creates space and without which it is impossible to see the anatomy of the mucosal folds. The telescope

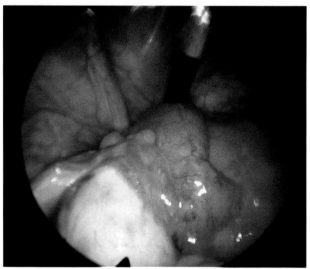

Fig. 4.5.2 Salpingoscopy.
The tube has been aligned with the laparoscope to bring the fimbriae and tubal ostium into view.

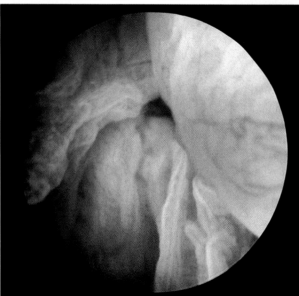

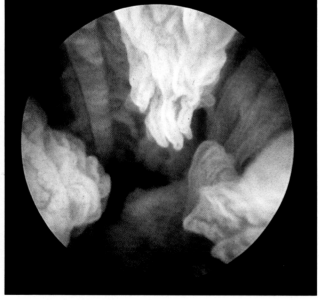

Fig. 4.5.3a–e Normal tubal mucosa.
a The tubal infundibulum showing the concentric arrangement of the folds.

b The tubal ampulla; three major folds can be seen with smaller minor folds between them.

is then advanced slowly and gently out of the sheath, under direct vision, into the tubal infundibulum where the major and minor folds can be easily seen (Fig. 4.5.3a).

In the normal tube the folds are well formed and parallel to each other and move freely in the distending fluid. The tubal lumen should be followed into the ampulla (Fig. 4.5.3b) by advancing the telescope and negotiating the bends with care. In the ampulla there are 4–6 major folds, each about 4 mm in height, with accessory folds arising from them. Between the major folds there are several minor folds approximately

1 mm in height. When the junction of the ampulla and isthmus is reached the major folds give way to three or four rounded folds 200–400 μm in height (Fig. 4.5.3c).

Using magnification, the vascular pattern of the capillaries in the ampullary mucosal folds (Fig. 4.5.3d) can be studied, but neither the cellular pattern nor the cilia are visible at this magnification. With experience, it is usually possible to follow the lumen of the tube as far as the isthmo-ampullary junction. Finally proximal tubal patency can be confirmed by chromopertubation with dilute methylene blue. The dye passes through the tube and stains the mucosa (Fig. 4.5.3e).

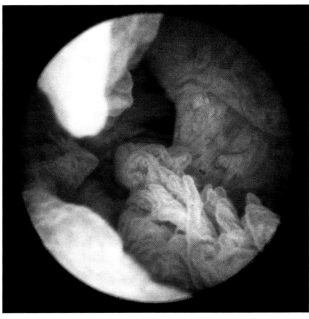

c The isthmo-ampullary junction; the minor folds can be seen running towards the isthmus.

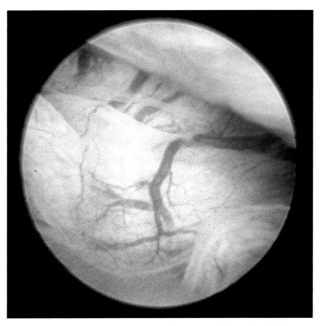

d At ×20 magnification, the vascular pattern of a major fold can be seen.

e Dilute methylene blue stains the mucosa of the ampullary folds.

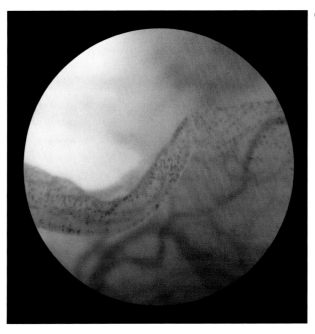

A hydrosalpinx must be mobilized if there are adhesions and then opened at the site of obstruction (Fig. 4.5.4) to permit introduction of the salpingoscope and inspection of the tubal mucosa. In some cases the mucosal folds are well preserved (Fig. 4.5.5) and these offer good results from tubal reconstructive surgery. In others, however, infection has resulted in flattening of the major folds, which are wide apart, or have

adhesions between them (Fig. 4.5.6). In these cases a successful outcome from surgery is most unlikely.

Flexible Salpingoscopy

An alternative technique uses a 3.4 mm flexible bronchoscope and an operating laparoscope. The uterus should

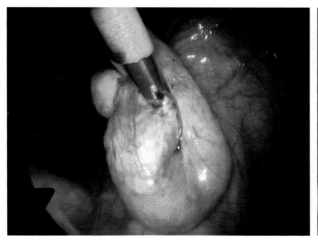

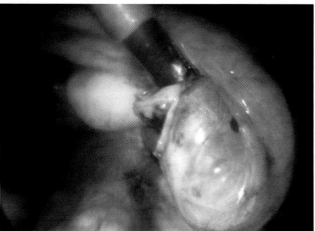

Fig. 4.5.4a & b Hydrosalpinx.
a The terminal end of the hydrosalpinx is held with atraumatic forceps.

b The hydrosalpinx has been opened to permit the introduction of a salpingoscope.

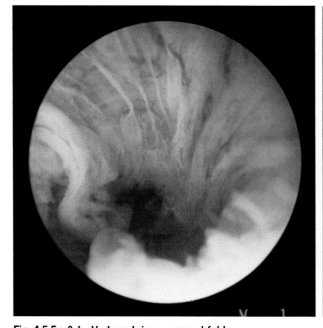

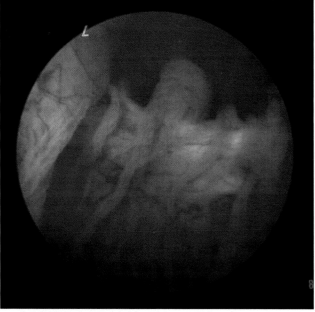

Fig. 4.5.5a & b Hydrosalpinx – normal folds.
a The major mucosal folds are well-preserved.

b Magnification demonstrates that the folds are normal.

be retroverted and rotated, as described for rigid salpingoscopy, to bring the fallopian tube onto its anterior aspect and align it with the laparoscope. The fimbriae are then grasped with fine flexible colon biopsy forceps and the tip of the telescope is inserted into the tube (Fig. 4.5.7a). The insufflating channel is connected to a saline infusion which is run freely. Unlike the rigid telescope whose focal length varies from zero to infinity, the focal length of the flexible telescope is 3 mm. It is impossible to see the tubal mucosa when it is in contact with the lens so there must always be a fluid filled space between the lens and the mucosa. The telescope must therefore be advanced very gently under laparoscopic vision as far as the isthmo-ampullary junction and the tube inspected as it is being withdrawn (Fig. 4.5.7 b) using the space in front of the lens to keep the

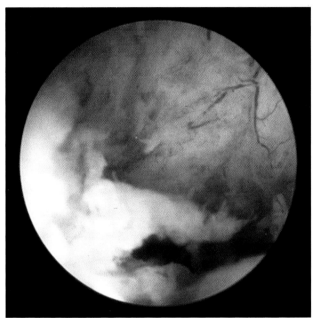

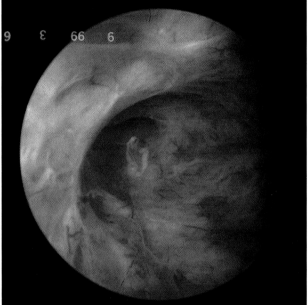

Fig. 4.5.6a–f Hydrosalpinx – damaged folds.
a The mucosal folds are irregular.

b Dense fibrous tissue is seen in the tubal wall.

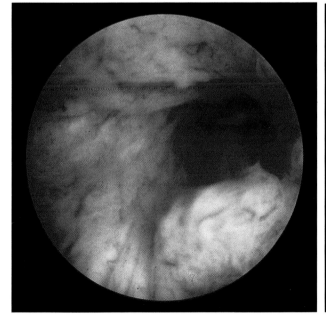

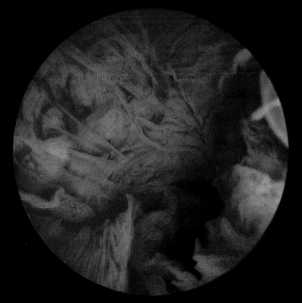

c The folds are conglutinated.

d An area of complete loss of fold pattern is seen.

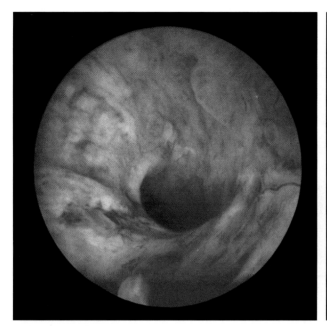

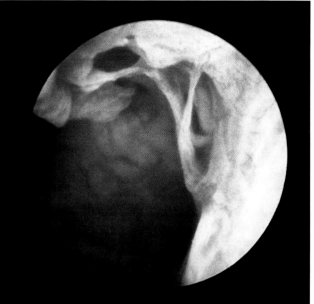

Fig. 4.5.6 continued.

e Fibrosis of the tubal wall and loss of the fold pattern.

f Fibrous adhesions are seen between the mucosal folds.

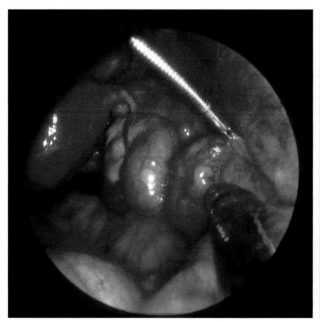

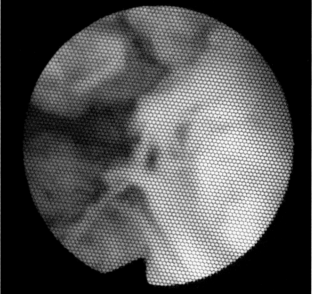

Fig. 4.5.7a & b Salpingoscopy.

a The fimbriae are held with fine forceps and the salpingoscope is entering the tubal ostium.

b Adhesions between the major folds of the ampulla seen through a flexible salpingoscope. (Courtesy of Dr Edgard Cornier.)

mucosal folds in focus. The hand movements to insert the telescope must be very fine to avoid damage to the tubal mucosa and for this reason considerable technical skill is required.

In theory the flexible telescope should be easier to steer along a tortuous tube but, in practice, the tube can be straightened by gentle traction and there is usually no difficulty in passing a rigid telescope along its full length. The rigid telescope with its rod lens

gives a clearer and brighter image with a wider field of vision and costs about one third as much as a flexible telescope.

Complications

Complications from salpingoscopy are rare. In addition to the recognized complications of laparoscopy, it is possible to damage the fimbriae with the forceps and cause minor bleeding or, possibly, adhesion formation. This has rarely been a problem but, nevertheless, it is preferable to introduce the telescope without grasping the fimbriae. The tube-holding forceps are designed to hold the tube without compressing it and so pressure damage is unlikely.

The most serious complication is damage to the tube and perforation of the tubal mucosa which can occur if the telescope is advanced blindly or if there are clumsy or rough movements of the telescope. The need for very gentle handling of the tube and instruments cannot be stressed too strongly. With these safeguards, there should be no significant complications from salpingoscopy.

Salpingoscopy at Tubal Reconstructive Surgery

In view of the relationship between the degree and extent of the lesions and the results of surgery in terms of pregnancy, salpingoscopy should be performed during reconstructive tubal surgery.

The tube should be mobilized by adhesiolysis and, if necessary, terminal salpingostomy carried out as in the standard performance of tubal reconstructive surgery. A microcolpohysteroscope with a diameter of 5.2 mm can then be inserted through the fimbrial opening and a saline infusion run freely through the insufflating channel to distend the tube. The mucosa is then examined from the infundibulum to the medial ampulla and its suitability for surgery assessed.

REFERENCES

Boer–Meisel, M.E., Te Velde, E.R., Habbema, J.D.F. & Kardaun, J.W.P.F. (1986) Predicting the pregnancy outcome in patients treated for hydrosalpinges: a light optical and scanning electron microscopy study. *British Journal of Obstetrics and Gynaecology*, **45**, 23–29.

Brosens, I., Boeckx, W., Delattin, Ph., Puttemans. P. & Vasquez, G. (1987) Salpingoscopy: a new pre-operative diagnostic tool in tubal infertility. *British Journal of Obstetrics and Gynaecology*, **94**, 768–773.

Brosens, I.A. & Vasquez, G. (1976) Fimbrial microbiopsy. *Journal of Reproductive Medicine*, **16**, 171–178.

Brundin, J., Dahlborn, M., Ahlberg–Ahre, E. & Lundberg, H.J. (1989) Radionuclide hysterosalpingography for measurement of human oviductal function. *International Journal of Gynecology and Obstetrics*, **28**, 53–59.

Chamberlain, G. & Carron-Brown, J. (1977) *Gynaecological Laparoscopy*. Royal College of Obstetricians and Gynaecologists. 105–121.

Cornier, E. (1982) La fibroscopie en gynecologie: la fibro-hysteroscopie et la fibrotuboscopie. *Nouvelle Presse Medicale*, **11**, 2841–2843.

Cornier, E. (1985) L'ampullosalpingoscopie per-coelioscopique. *Journal de Gynecologie, Obstetrique et Biologie de la Reproduction*, **14**, 459–466.

Cumming, D.C. & Taylor, P.J. (1979) Historical predictability of abnormal laparoscopic findings in infertile women. *Journal of Reproductive Medicine*, **23**, 295–298.

David, M.P., Ben-Zwi, D. & Langer, L. (1981) Tubal intramural polyps and their relationship to infertility. *Fertility and Sterility*, **35**, 526–531.

DeCherney, A.H., Kort, H., Barney, J.B. & De Vore, R. (1980) Increased pregnancy rate with oil-soluble hysterosalpingography. *Fertility and Sterility*, **33**, 407–410.

Donnez, J., Langerock, S., Lecart, C.I. & Thomas, K. (1982) Incidence of pathological factors not revealed by hysterosalpingography but disclosed by laparoscopy in 500 infertile women. *European Journal of Obstetrics and Gynecology and Reproductive Biology*, **13**, 369–375.

Hamou, J.E. (1980) Hysteroscopie et microhysteroscopie avec un instrument nouveau: le microhysteroscope. *Endoscopic Gynecology*, **2**, 131.

Henry-Suchet, J., Tesquiter, L., Pez, J.P. & Loffredo, V. (1984) Prognostic value of tuboscopy vs hysterosalpingography before tuboplasty. *Journal of Reproductive Medicine*, **29**, 602–612.

Iturralde, M. & Venter, F.F. (1981) Hysterosalpingo-radionuclide scintigraphy (HERS). *Seminars in Nuclear Medicine*, **XI**, 301.

Lindemann, H.J. (1971) Eine neue untersuchungstmethode für die Hysteroskopie. *Endoscopy*, **3**, 194–199.

Marshak, R.H., Rode, C.S. & Goldberger, M.A. (1950) Hysterography and hysterosalpingography. *Surgery, Gynecology and Obstetrics*, **91**, 182–192.

McCalley, M.G., Braunstein, P., Stone, S., Henderson, P. & Egbert, R. (1985) Radionuclide hysterosalpingography for evaluation of tubal patency. *Journal of Nuclear Medicine*, **26**, 868–874.

Measday, B. (1960) An analysis of the complications of hysterosalpingography. *Journal of Obstetrics and Gynaecology of the British Empire*, **67**, 663–667.

Mohri, T., Mohri, K. & Yamadori, F. (1970) Tubaloscope. Flexible glassfiber endoscope for intratubal observation. *Endoscopy*, **4**, 226–230.

Palmer, A. (1960) Ethiodol hysterosalpingography for the treatment of infertility. *Fertility and Sterility*, **11**, 311–315.

Phillips, J.M., Keith, D., Keith, L., Hulka, J. & Hulka, B. (1975) Survey of gynecologic laparoscopy for 1974. *Journal of Reproductive Medicine*, **15**, 45–50.

Stumph, P.G. & March, C.M. (1980) Febrile morbidity following hysterosalpingography: identification of risk factors and recommendations for prophylaxis. *Fertility and Sterility*, **33**, 487–492.

Westrom, L. & Märdh, P.A. (1980) Reproductive events after salpingitis. In *Sexually Transmitted Diseases. Status Report. NIAID Study Group*. pp.43–54. NIH Publications Ltd.

5   THE TREATMENT OF TUBAL INFERTILITY

5.1 TUBAL AND OVARIAN MICROSURGERY
Willy Boeckx

Introduction

Although retention of function has always been an important factor in gynaecological surgery, the presence of an ovary and tube on each side of the uterus has frequently been used as a pretext for performing unilateral oöphorectomy or salpingectomy for benign disease. However any uterine, tubal or ovarian surgery can lead to the formation of adhesions, ovarian failure and tubal dysfunction with subsequent subfertility or sterility. A full assessment of the indications and techniques of pelvic surgery may prevent such loss of fertility.

Instruments for Microsurgery

Microsurgery involves the use of magnification to enable delicate surgery to be performed with minimal tissue trauma and accurate reconstruction of the different organs. Adequate training in the techniques involved is vitally important.

High Power Magnification
High power magnification can be obtained with an operating microscope with twin optics to allow 'team work' so that the assistant can hold tissues and achieve bipolar haemostasis whilst the surgeon carries out sharp dissection. There should also be a video attachment for the training of other members of staff. An electric foot-controlled zoom lens with a magnification from $\times 8$–$\times 25$ is essential for fine tubal and ovarian surgery, but preliminary lysis of adhesions deep in the pelvis is better performed using a Keeler operation loupe giving $\times 6$ magnification.

Micro-Electric Surgical Procedures
Micro-electric surgical procedures play an important role in tubal and ovarian surgery. A low intensity cutting coagulating current using a finger-controlled handle should be used to activate a 0.2 mm insulated needle to divide adhesions, perform salpingostomy and incise the ovarian capsule. Haemostasis and coagulation of peritoneal endometriotic deposits can be achieved using bipolar current applied with fine jewellers forceps which limit the diameter of the burned area.

The Operating Instruments
The operating instruments for microsurgery include microscissors, fine suture-cutting scissors, microforceps and spring-loaded microneedle holders, which are used for suture-tying. Fine 8/0 nylon sutures on a round bodied needle should be used for all tubal surgery and the ovarian capsule, whereas thicker 5/0 polyethylene is suitable for stay sutures and for suturing the ovarian stroma. Glass hooks which do not conduct electrical current are used to retract organs without causing trauma.

During the procedure a silastic sheet should be placed on top of the pelvic pack to act as an 'intra-abdominal operating table' on which the tubes and ovaries can lie. This provides a smooth non-traumatic surface and prevents encapsulation of cotton wool fibres from the packs. Also the abdomen and pelvis should be continuously irrigated with warm Hartmann's solution throughout the operation to prevent the peritoneum and fimbriae drying, tissues sticking together, and blood clotting, and a sump drain is inserted to provide continuous drainage of the pouch of Douglas.

Preparation of the Patient

The patient should be admitted on the day prior to surgery and be prepared for laparotomy. Antibiotics are not used prophylactically but are given if there are specific indications in the postoperative period. During the operation an indwelling urethral catheter should be inserted to keep the bladder empty, and if the procedure includes reversal of sterilization, 20 ml of methylene blue is injected into the uterus through a Rubins' catheter to identify the site of tubal occlusion. A vaginal pack is inserted to lift the uterus and improve accessibility of the tubes.

Incision and Exposure

A transverse skin incision should be employed and the anterior rectus sheath is then incised above the pubic bone (Cherney, 1941). The rectus muscle is then separated from the os pubis and retracted cranially for about 7 cm. This is followed by a transverse incision of the peritoneum taking care to avoid the deep epigastric vessels, which allows easy access to the fallopian tubes and ovaries. The small bowel is packed into the upper abdominal cavity, a plastic wound protector is inserted, and a Kirschner four bladed retractor is used to expose the pelvic organs. An irrigation system is then installed to allow continuous flow of Hartmann's solution at 37°C which is simultaneously drained from the pouch of Douglas.

Adhesions

Adhesions are not common in patients undergoing reversal of sterilization, but if present, two glass hooks should be used to stretch them and facilitate their division using unipolar electrosurgery. When larger blood vessels are encountered, bipolar coagulation must be used before transecting them and restoring the normal anatomy. The uterus, ovary and tubes can now be lifted out of the abdomen and the pouch of Douglas is packed with wet abdominal packs. The silastic sheet is then placed under the ovaries and fallopian tubes to stabilize them and to prevent tissue trauma and the microscope is brought into position.

Reversal of Sterilization

Tubo-Tubal Anastomosis

Most modern laparoscopic sterilization methods occlude the fallopian tube at the isthmus or isthmo-ampullary junction and to reverse the operation the occluded segment must be completely removed as follows.

1. The tube must first be transected proximally and distally to the site of occlusion (Fig. 5.1.1a) The overlying serosa is incised with unipolar diathermy until the blood supply of the outer layer of the circular muscle coat is visible. The circular muscle coat, which is about 0.5 mm thick, and the mucosa, are then transected with microscissors (Fig. 5.1.1b); these are used in preference to electrosurgery to avoid thermal damage to the delicate mucosa, which is inspected under high power magnification when it is exposed (Fig. 5.1.1c). The methylene blue dye will be seen to stain the mucosal folds and the circular muscle layers, and the direction of a jet of warm Hartmann's solution into the tubal lumen should produce gentle dilatation of the tube indicating that normal mucosa has been reached. If the lumen fails to dilate, further resection of small tubal segments should be performed until normal mucosa, recognizable by the capillary vessels in the mucosal folds, is found.

2. A blunt metal probe with a groove is introduced through the fimbriae and ampulla to the site of tubal obstruction (Fig. 5.1.1d). A 0.4 mm polyethylene catheter is placed in the groove until it locks into the narrow constriction of the groove. Next, the metal probe is withdrawn thereby introducing the polyethylene splint into the distal part of the tube. About 5 cm of the proximal part of the splint is then fed into the uterus, which is facilitated by stretching the proximal segment of the tube (Fig. 5.1.1e). This splint helps to align both segments of the tube and avoids kinking at the site of anastomosis.

3. The cut ends of the tube are approximated with a single 5/0 polyethylene stitch placed in the mesentery close to the tubal muscle (Fig. 5.1.1f). This stay suture helps to prevent tension on the microsurgical suture line. Isthmo-isthmic tubal anastomosis is then performed with atraumatic 8/0 nylon sutures on a round bodied 140 micron needle (Fig. 5.1.1g). This stitch should take a relatively large bite of the circular muscle coat but care should be taken not to include the mucosa as an ectopic pregnancy can result from distortion of the mucosal fold pattern. The first 8/0 nylon suture is placed at the mesenteric or 6 o'clock position (Fig. 5.1.1h). The second and third stitches are placed medially and laterally to the first stitch respectively and, when the posterior wall has been repaired, further stitches should be inserted to approximate the circular coat, ensuring that the mucosa is not included in the suture. If anastomosis has to be performed on tubal segments of unequal size, the distance between the stitches is closer than normal in the narrow diameter segment and at a normal distance in the larger diameter portion. The distance between the stitches should be approximately 0.2–0.3 mm.

4. After completion of the anastomosis of the circular muscle coat the overlying serosa is repaired using a running suture of 8/0 nylon if there is no tension on the suture line (Fig. 5.1.1i). When there is tension on the suture line, interrupted sutures are used. Inversion of the serosal edge should result in a smooth surface without haematoma or petechiae (Fig. 5.1.1j), and meticulous approximation of the serosa using high power magnification avoids postoperative adhesions. When the anastomosis has been completed, the polyethylene splint is removed through the fimbrial end of the tube.

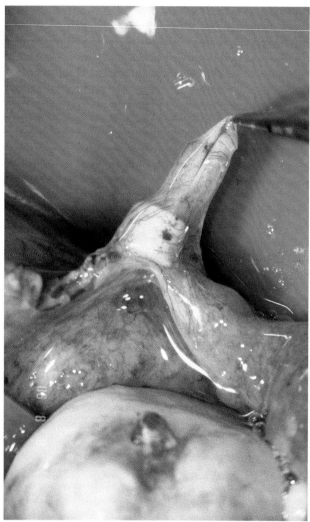

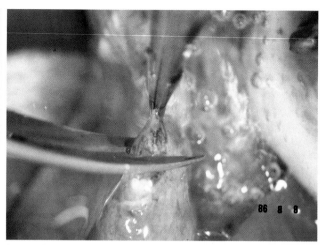

b The muscularis and mucosa are being transected with microscissors.

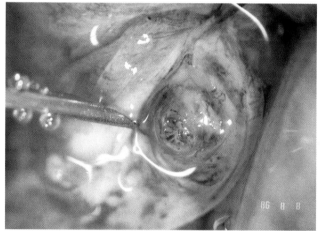

Fig. 5.1.1 a–j Reversal of sterilization – tubo-tubal anastomosis.
a Tubal sterilization has been performed with a fallope ring. The apex of the loop has been stretched to display the site of occlusion.

c The isthmic mucosa is inspected under high-power magnification to ensure that normal mucosa has been reached.

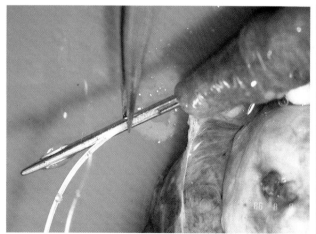

d A metal probe has been inserted through the fimbriae and protrudes from the distal segment of the isthmus. The polythene splint has been fed into the groove.

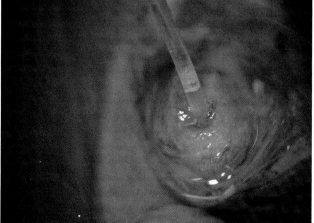

e The splint has been inserted into the proximal segment of the isthmus.

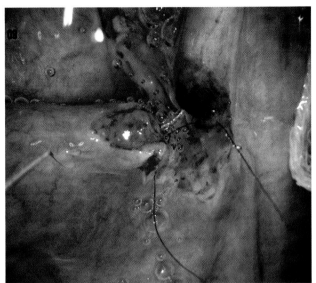

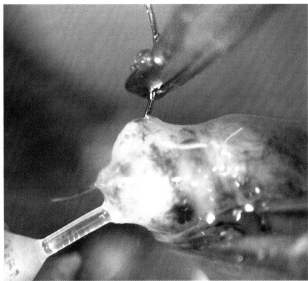

f A stay suture of 5/0 prolene has been inserted into the tubal mesentery to approximate the cut ends of the isthmus.

g The myosalpinx is being sutured with 8/0 nylon; the sutures must not penetrate the mucosa.

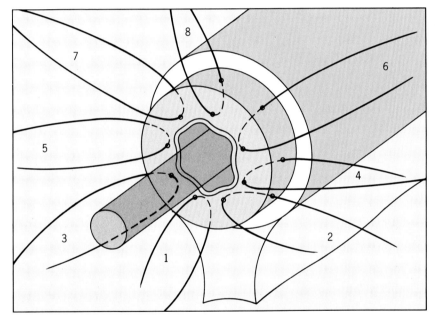

h The order of placement of the sutures in the myosalpinx.

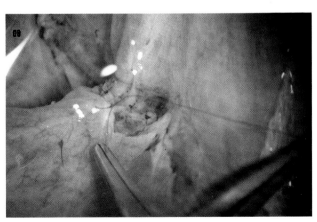

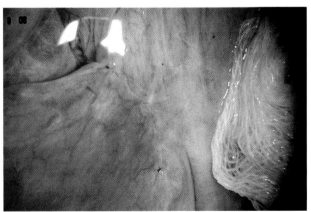

i Repair of the serosa with continuous 8/0 nylon suture.

j Completion of the operation with inversion of the serosal edge.

Tubo-Cornual Anastomosis

When sterilization has been carried out by electro-coagulation or when tubo-cornual anastomosis has to be performed, there is usually a larger defect in the tubal mesentery (Fig. 5.1.2a). In these cases the distal segment of the fallopian tube must be mobilized, opened, and approximated to the uterine cornu before starting the anastomosis (Fig. 5.1.2b).

A longitudinal incision is made in the myometrium of the uterine cornu and the muscle is retracted to expose the intramural portion of the tube, following which the tube is isolated by circumcising the myometrium using electrosurgery. When the site of occlusion has been identified, the circular muscle is cut segmentally with microscissors under high power magnification (Fig. 5.1.2c). The blood supply of the intramural portion is then carefully assessed to evaluate the quality of the mucosa, and the dissection is complete when well-vascularized mucosal folds are encountered.

A splint is then inserted as described for tubo-tubal anastomosis and the circular muscle coat is sutured avoiding the mucosa (Fig. 5.1.2d). The mesenteric stitch is inserted first and subsequent stitches are added on alternate sides to gradually anastomose the posterior and then the anterior wall of the tube. If bleeding occurs, vasopressin should be injected to produce vasoconstriction and reduce bleeding into the operative field. The serosa is then sutured with interrupted stitches (Fig. 5.1.2e), the edge being inverted to produce smooth apposition of the serosa and to avoid leaving a raw surface which could become a site of adhesion formation.

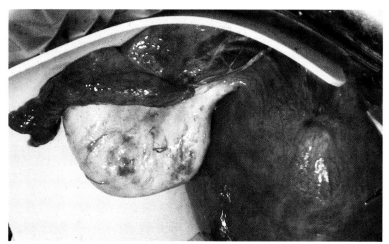

Fig. 5.1.2a–e Reversal of sterilization – tubo-cornual anastomosis.
a Sterilization has been performed by tubal coagulation which has resulted in a large defect in the tubal mesentery.

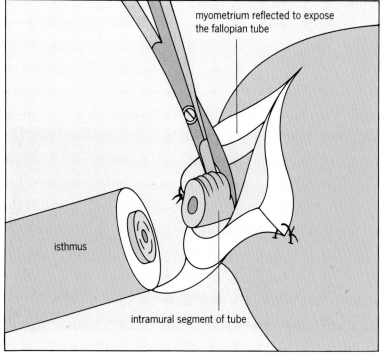

myometrium reflected to expose the fallopian tube

isthmus

intramural segment of tube

b Preparation of the distal tube and cornu before commencing the anastomosis.

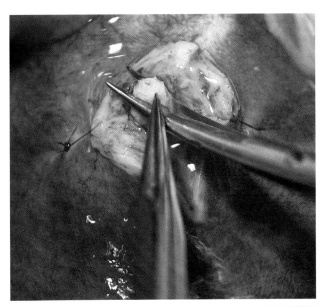

c The myometrium has been incised with unipolar diathermy, and the circular muscle of the intramural segment and the mucosa is being divided with scissors.

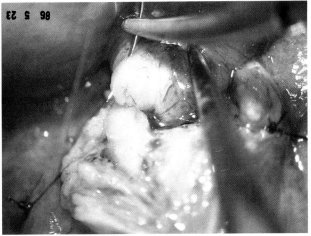

d The myosalpinx is being sutured with 8/0 nylon, avoiding the mucosa.

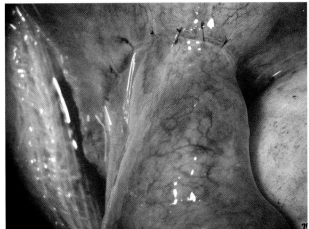

e Interrupted sutures in the serosa complete the operation.

Cuff Salpingostomy

The most suitable condition to benefit from micro-surgical salpingostomy is thin-walled hydrosalpinx simplex.

1. The abdominal incision and exposure of the fallopian tubes are performed as described earlier (see page 5.2) (Fig. 5.1.3a).

2. The site of the distal occlusion of the fallopian tube is inspected under high power magnification (Fig. 5.1.3b) and where the superficial blood vessels converge, which is not at the anatomical apex of the fallopian tube, the tube is incised to create a new ostium. Electrosurgery is used to make a Y-shaped incision (Fig. 5.1.3c) with three mucosal flaps which, when everted, expose the tubal mucosa.

3. The expanded hydrosalpinx will collapse as soon as the tube is opened and two glass hooks should be inserted to stretch the hydrosalpinx walls (Fig. 5.1.3d) whilst an insulated unipolar electrode is used to incise the serosa, circular muscle coat and mucosa. The incisions must be made parallel to the blood vessels or, when possible, parallel to the mucosal folds in the tubal lumen.

4. The circular muscle coat and mucosa are next everted using the two glass hooks (Fig. 5.1.3e). Care must be taken to avoid grasping the delicate mucosa with forceps which should only be used to hold the cut surface of the circular muscle coat (Fig. 5.1.3f). After completely everting the tubal mucosa, the cone-shaped opening of the newly-formed salpingostomy should remain open (Fig. 5.1.3g). The mucosa is then stitched to the serosa using 8/0 nylon sutures to bury the cut surface as before and avoid adhesion formation.

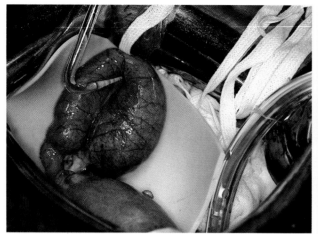

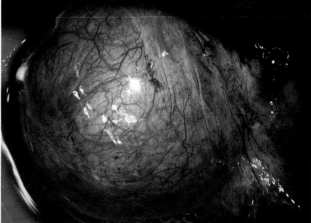

Fig. 5.1.3a–g Cuff salpingostomy.
a A thin-walled hydrosalpinx has been displayed on the silicone sheet using glass hooks.

b The site of occlusion is examined under high-power magnification.

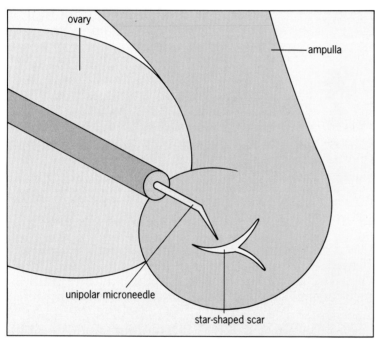

c The site of the incision is recognized by the star-shaped scar on the terminal ampulla. The unipolar microneedle is used to make a cruciate incision.

d Glass hooks stretching the neo-ostium.

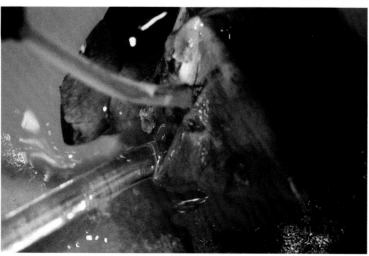

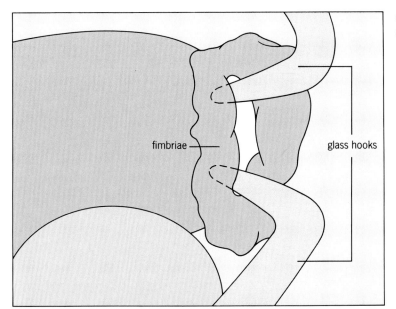

e Glass hooks everting the circular muscle and mucosa.

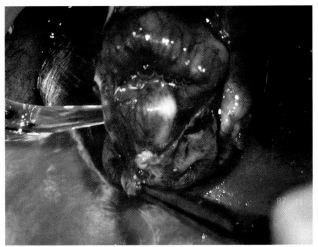

f Glass hooks evert the tube while the forceps hold only the muscularis, avoiding the serosa and mucosa.

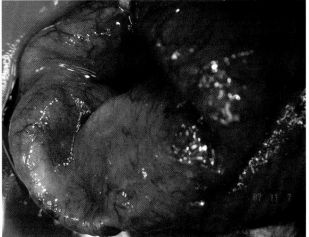

g Completed cuff salpingostomy.

Microsurgery for Ovarian Endometriosis

In extensive long-standing ovarian endometriosis, there are frequently dense adhesions between the ovarian surface and the surrounding organs such as the sigmoid colon or the small bowel and these should first be removed (Fig. 5.1.4a). When the adhesions are thick, the small blood vessels must be coagulated with bipolar forceps before excising the adhesions with unipolar electrosurgery. The fallopian tube can then be mobilized. The fimbrial mucosa in patients with endometriosis is usually found to be healthy. The ovary can next be elevated and stabilized on the silastic sheet.

The ovarian cortex is first incised elliptically with the micro-electrosurgery needle to expose the endometrioma (Fig. 5.1.4b), and then the healthy ovarian cortex and stroma are retracted with two glass hooks, and the pseudocapsule of the endometrioma is removed (Fig. 5.1.4c). The plane of dissection can be identified between the ovarian endometrioma and the healthy ovary using microscissors and ×8 magnification. Rupture of the endometrioma can rarely be avoided but thorough washing of the chocolate cyst with warm Hartmann's solution and further aspiration of the fluid will remove the spilled contents. Steady traction on the cyst wall accompanied by microscissor dissection allows the plane of dissection to be followed deep into the ovarian hilus so that the cyst can be completely removed.

After bipolar coagulation of the small blood vessels in the ovarian stroma, the two halves of the ovary should be brought together with inverted stitches of

5/0 polyethylene (Fig. 5.1.4d), which are inserted into the base of the stroma of one half of the ovary and brought out close to the ovarian surface (Fig. 5.1.4e). The suture can be continued close to the surface of the other half and carried down to the deepest part of the ovary before being tied. Progressive suturing allows the reconstruction of the normal anatomical shape of the ovary.

The ovarian cortex should be finally closed with a running suture of 8/0 nylon (Fig. 5.1.4f), inverting the cut edge of the ovarian incision to produce a smooth ovarian surface.

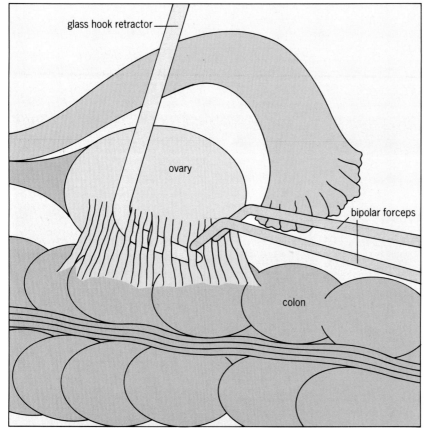

Fig. 5.1.4a–f Microsurgery for ovarian endometriosis.
a Division of adhesions between the ovary and large bowel.

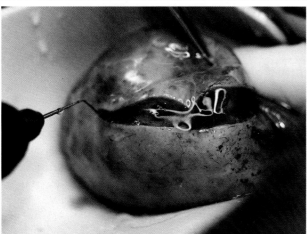

b An elliptical incision is made in the ovarian cortex to expose the endometrioma.

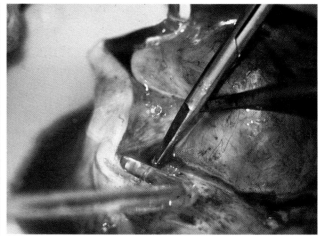

c The pseudocapsule of the endometrioma is removed by sharp dissection and peeling it from the ovarian stroma.

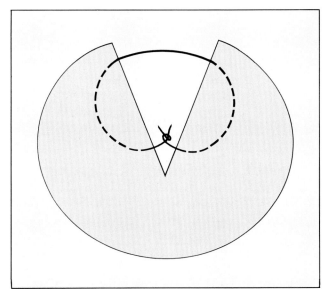

d Inverted deep sutures are placed in the ovarian tissue commencing deep in the ovary.

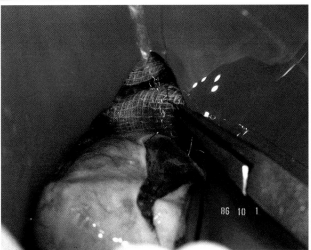

e The suture has been brought out near the ovarian capsule.

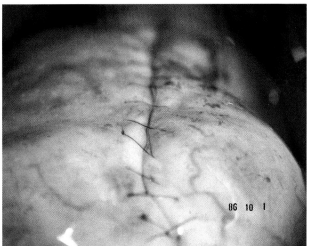

f The ovarian capsule is closed with a continuous 8/0 nylon suture accurately approximating and inverting the edge.

5.2 LAPAROSCOPIC SURGERY
Thierry Vancaillie

Operative laparoscopic surgery has developed as an extension of diagnostic laparoscopy during the last 20 years. A relatively small number of surgeons in Europe and North America have demonstrated that it has some advantages over conventional pelvic surgery, the main ones being that there are fewer postoperative complications and ileus is unlikely to occur. Some surgeons (Semm, 1982) have replaced laparotomy by laparoscopy in up to 80% of cases, reducing hospital costs by 50% and community costs significantly because of the shorter recovery time (Levine, 1985). Nevertheless the introduction of surgery into gynaecological endoscopy has occurred some 50 years after similar developments in urological surgery and it has still to gain universal acceptance in the speciality.

Technical Skill

Extensive laparoscopic surgery may take several hours to perform, so operating schedules may have to be altered accordingly and nursing staff re-educated to accept the value of this form of surgery. More specifically, such surgery demands a much higher degree of skill than that required by diagnostic laparoscopy and simple operative procedures such as sterilization. In addition, surgeons must learn new techniques, the use of new instruments and must understand the limits of laparoscopic surgery.

The surgeon should be an experienced laparoscopist, preferably with a background in microsurgical techniques. His initial training should be with the use of inert models but practical demonstrations and video films are also of value. 'Hands on' training with an experienced laparoscopist to master the techniques is essential. The development of technical skill should commence with simple procedures such as division of fine adhesions before proceeding to more extensive adhesiolysis, resection of ovarian cysts, salpingectomy and laparoscopic tubal reconstructive surgery.

Maintaining an Adequate Pneumoperitoneum

Maintaining an adequate pneumoperitoneum with a safe intra-abdominal pressure throughout the procedure is essential. Multiple trocars with frequent changes of instruments lead to loss of gas which cannot readily be replaced using a manually operated instrument. An electronic insufflator keeps the intra-abdominal pressure at a pre-set level and requires no further monitoring.

Sutures

Sutures may occasionally be required to control haemorrhage or, rarely, to reconstruct organs. A slip knot based on the Roeder loop can be applied to a cut pedicle and should be part of the normal instrumentation. Duplicating microsurgical suture techniques is technically impossible. The finest suture available for endoscopic surgery is 3/0 and the needle must be strong enough to be used with laparoscopic needle holders. However, the most important limitation in fine suturing techniques is the working distance between the surgeon's hands and the tissue, which is usually 35 cm or more. This limits the ability to perform delicate procedures. Sutures, other than for haemostasis, will soon be replaced by tissue welding techniques such as those currently being used for everting a salpingostomy.

Thermal Control of Intraperitoneal Bleeding

Thermal control of intraperitoneal bleeding is essential and the methods available include unipolar and bipolar electrocoagulation and thermal coagulation. Unipolar electrocoagulation is potentially hazardous due to the unpredictable return pathway of the current towards the dispersive electrode (Rioux, 1977). Careful use of the newer, better designed, instruments has virtually eliminated complications which were common in the early seventies and which were partly contributed to by the inexperience of the surgeons. Bipolar coagulation is safer (Palmer, 1974) but does not allow cutting. The current flows between the electrodes, which are usually the blades of tissue forceps. There may be damage outside the operative field by direct transmission of heat, but other serious complications can occur when two different electrical generators, one for

unipolar current and the other for bipolar current, are connected to the patient. In this case the current generated at the bipolar instrument may be attracted to the dispersive electrode of the other generator and cause inadvertent damage to other structures at a distance from the operative site and outside the visual field of the surgeon. Alternatively, thermal coagulators may be used. These apply heat at 80–120°C for a preset time of 20–40 seconds, producing a tissue response similar to that of bipolar electrocoagulation but with a slower action and less chance of remote tissue damage by the elimination of direct transfer of electrical energy. The use of laser for intraperitoneal surgery will be discussed in Section 5.3.

Peritoneal Irrigation

Peritoneal irrigation during and at the completion of the operation removes blood and debris and also helps to prevent reformation of adhesions. An irrigating pump may be used to irrigate physiological or heparinized Ringer's solution during the operation, which may be followed by a corticosteroid solution or dextran instillation at the completion.

Physical Fatigue

Physical fatigue during lengthy operative procedures may be combatted by adjusting the table height and by altering the Trendelenburg tilt. Video cameras also help the surgeon to operate either directly off the screen or through the lens using a beam splitter. The modern chip camera, with its light weight and improved definition, has been a major factor in the development of this type of surgery, by allowing the assistant to manipulate tissues more accurately and making the supervision of trainees safer.

Proceeding to Laparotomy

Both the surgeon and patient must be prepared to proceed to laparotomy if complications arise or if the condition is not amenable to laparoscopic surgery. However, with increasing experience, the change in operative techniques should become less common but may always be necessary if there is extensive fibrosis involving the bowel and retroperitoneal space.

Elective Surgery

The general principles of endoscopic surgery are similar to those of conventional surgery but are subject to certain limitations imposed by the reduced mobility of the ancillary instruments. The surgeon must first ensure adequate access to the pelvic cavity. In patients who have had previous abdominal surgery, adhesions between the omentum and abdominal wall are common and must be lysed to obtain unobstructed access. Adhesions prevent upward displacement of the bowel, thus increasing the operative difficulty.

Adhesiolysis

The simplest laparoscopic operation is adhesiolysis, which should always begin at the anterior abdominal

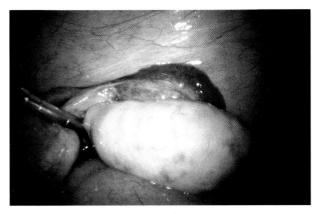

Fig. 5.2.1 Anteluxation of the right ovary.
A probe has been placed beneath the right ovary which is moved upwards and laterally, while the uterus is displaced towards the ipsilateral ovarian fossa.

wall or pelvic brim and progress downwards towards the pouch of Douglas. The scissors, electrical needle or laser must always approach the operation site at a perpendicular angle which is achieved by manipulating the uterus, using multiple trocars to vary the angle of approach and placing traction on the adhesion to be lysed.

As in conventional surgery, it is essential to assess the exact anatomy by manipulating the pelvic organs to inspect them in detail (Fig. 5.2.1). During adhesiolysis the edge of the peritoneum, or other normal tissue to which the adhesion is attached, should be located, to allow accurate reconstruction. An awareness of the possible organs underlying the adhesion is essential, particularly if electrical or thermal energy is being used, to prevent damage to the bowel, ureter or blood vessels. When, for example, an adhesion attaches the appendix to the fallopian tube (Fig. 5.2.2a), the incision to free the tube must be made along the tubal serosa (Fig. 5.2.2b) and not half-way between the organs. Fig. 5.2.2c shows the tube was abnormal with hydrosalpinx; much of the infundibulum is absent and there are adhesions between the tube and the appendix. In this case, however, it was unnecessary to correct the anatomy as the contralateral tube was apparently normal.

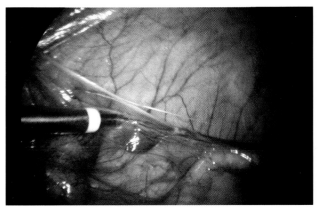

a

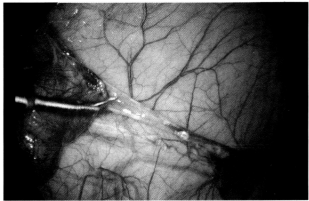

b

c

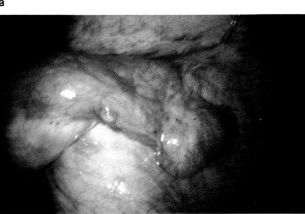

Fig. 5.2.2a–c Adhesion between the right fallopian tube and the appendix.

a Fine bipolar forceps are being used to coagulate the vessels in the adhesion prior to transection.

b Microscissors are being used to divide the adhesion along the edge of its tubal insertion.

c The tube is abnormal with distal blockage and hydrosalpinx. The ovary is lying high in the pelvis, and the infundibulum is deficient and the infundibulopelvic ligament is absent. Because of the absence of the tubal infundibulum, this hydrosalpinx was not corrected surgically.

Traction on adhesions, using flat forceps, aids accurate dissection (Fig. 5.2.3) and allows the scissors to reach the section line at a right angle and the adhesion to be divided along the surface of the ovary. Adhesions between the ovary and small bowel may result from pelvic inflammatory or bowel disease and can be divided safely using bipolar coagulation and scissors (Fig. 5.2.4).

Salpingostomy

The expert laparoscopist can extend the range of laparoscopic operative procedures to include tubal reconstructive surgery which can produce results equivalent to those of open microsurgery. Again, detailed morphological assessment is essential and an accurate evaluation of adhesions between the ovary and tube is imperative. Equally important is accurate location and identification of the tubo-ovarian ligament lying in the free edge of the mesosalpinx. This ligament contains a terminal artery which supplies the tubal infundibulum and accidental injury to it will result in necrosis and irreversible damage to the infundibulum.

When chronic pelvic inflammatory disease results in dense adhesions and hydrosalpinx (Fig. 5.2.5a), the surgeon must first perform a complete salpingo-ovariolysis followed by chromopertubation with dilute methylene blue to demonstrate proximal tubal patency and distend the tube. This highlights the star-shaped scar of the occluded infundibulum (Fig. 5.2.5b). If there is proximal tubal obstruction, laparoscopic surgery should be abandoned and tubal reconstructive surgery performed by laparotomy.

Following adhesiolysis, the scar on the occluded infundibulum is gradually incised by making multiple shallow cuts along its full length (Fig. 5.2.5c). This

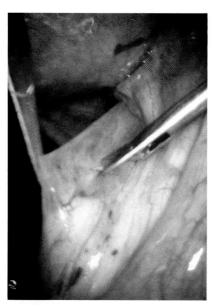

Fig. 5.2.3a & b Adhesion between the right ovary and the broad ligament.
a Flat forceps have grasped the adhesion and put it under tension in such a way that the scissors reach it at a right angle.

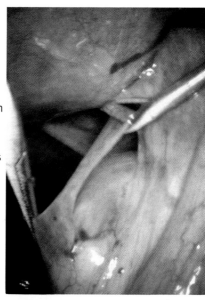

b The adhesion is being divided with scissors close to the ovarian surface and ovarian ligament.

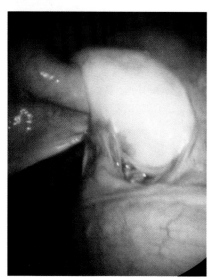

Fig. 5.2.4a & b Adhesion between the right ovary and the ileum.
The patient complained of pelvic pain.
a The site of the adhesion corresponds to the site of a possible Meckel's diverticulum.

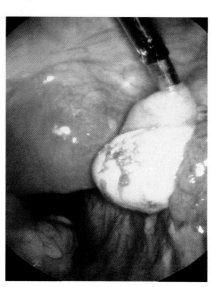

b Adhesiolysis was performed using bipolar coagulation and scissors. There was no apparent pathology in the ovary or bowel.

prevents premature perforation of the hydrosalpinx and its possible collapse. Next the tubal mucosa is inspected by salpingoscopy through a small incision in the terminal tube.

The incision of the scar is then completed (Fig. 5.2.5d), following which the edges of the opened tube are everted without suturing by heating the serosal surface to 60°C using endothermy, bipolar coagulation or defocused laser at a distance of approximately 5–10 mm from the distal edge. This causes the tissue to blanch and retract so that the tube everts and the neostium remains open (Fig. 5.2.5e). The blanching of the serosal surface of the infundibulum should be limited to the minimum necessary to obtain optimal eversion. Extensive blanching, which is a form of coagulation, may result in fibrosis of the tissue, reducing its mobility and possibly causing phimosis of the tube.

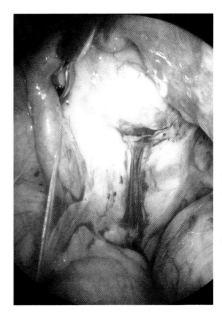

Fig. 5.2.5a–e The sequelae of pelvic inflammatory disease.

a The medial aspect of the left ovary and the left isthmus are seen. The left ampulla is covered with dense adhesions, and the distended infundibulum of a right hydrosalpinx is evident.

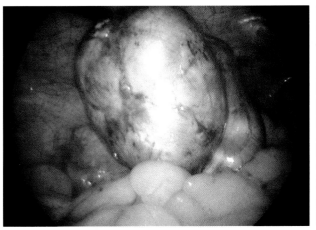

b The left tube has been freed from adhesions, and the ampulla is distended with methylene blue. The cruciate scar of the occluded infundibulum is seen.

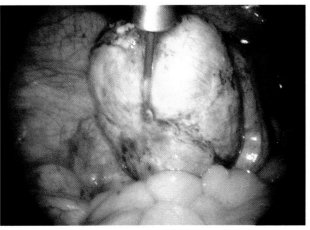

c The scar of the left hydrosalpinx is incised by making multiple shallow cuts with a monopolar needle electrode.

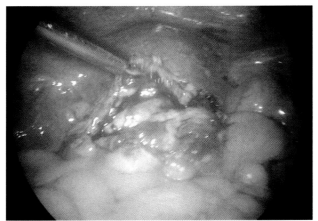

d The incision of the scar has been completed. There is loss of most of the mucosal folds of the infundibulum.

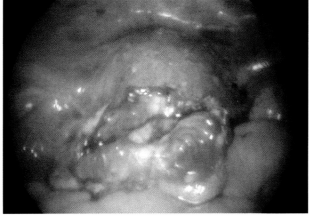

e The serosa has been blanched with bipolar forceps 5 mm from the incision line. The resultant retraction of the serosa everts the tube.

Cysts in the mesosalpinx may distort the fallopian tube and restrict its mobility. Fig. 5.2.6a shows a 6 cm cyst in the left mesosalpinx which should first be punctured (Fig. 5.2.6b) so that the tube can be accurately defined. The lateral aspect of the mesosalpinx is then incised to allow easy extraction of the cyst (Fig. 5.2.6c).

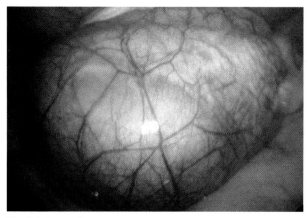

Fig. 5.2.6a–c Paraoöphoron cyst.

a The left mesosalpinx is distended by a 6 cm paraoöphoron cyst.

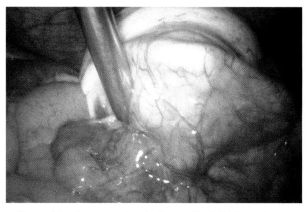

b The cyst has been punctured, allowing the left tube to be identified.

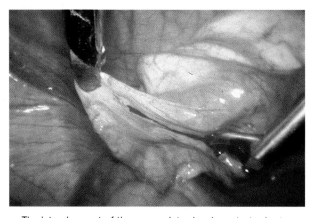

c The lateral aspect of the mesosalpinx has been incised prior to extraction of the cyst.

Emergency Surgery

Laparoscopy can be used as a mode of access for the diagnosis and treatment of a number of acute gynaecological conditions. The most important of these are pelvic inflammatory disease, tubal pregnancy and torsion of the adnexa. Even experienced physicians may misinterpret the symptoms in up to 40% of patients presenting with acute or subacute pelvic pain and consequently offer inappropriate treatment. Endoscopy should therefore be considered as essential in the management of the acute abdomen, as prompt and adequate treatment may salvage the tube and prevent or reduce the risk of subsequent infertility.

Acute Pelvic Inflammatory Disease

In patients with suspected pelvic inflammatory disease it is important to confirm the diagnosis and to determine the extent of the disease. In patients with minimal changes, the tubes may be only slightly oedematous with very small amounts of exudate in the cul-de-sac. The diagnosis may be made from a complete examination of the abdomen where the frequent occurrence of perihepatic adhesions (Fitz-Hugh-Curtis syndrome) will suggest gonococcal or chlamydial infection (Fig. 5.2.7). Sampling of the intratubal fluid by brush rather than by cotton swabs may yield better results due to richer cell sampling but, whichever technique is used, it is important to introduce the sampling device into the tubal lumen beyond the infundibulum, opening the tubal ostium if necessary to gain access. Aspirates of the exudate in the cul-de-sac yield little useful information and should not, therefore, be performed routinely.

When there is extensive pelvic inflammatory disease it is important to ascertain whether or not the ovaries are involved in the infective process with associated abscess formation. Laparoscopy with dissection of the adhesions will resolve the question. Drainage of the abscess may be all that is required and may prevent unnecessary oöphorectomy.

The principle of debridement for pelvic inflammatory disease is similar to that for other parts of the body. The aim is to remove all debris, fibrinous deposits and exudate so as to obtain a clean pelvis. The tissues are vascular, so only blunt dissection should be used or there may be bleeding which can be difficult to control. Sharp dissection may be necessary to divide multiple old adhesions, but should be used with extreme caution. After evacuating pus or exudate, the pelvic cavity, including the tubal lumen, must be rinsed profusely.

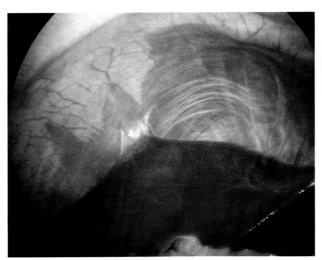

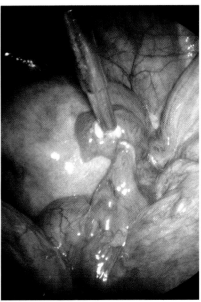

b A cotton swab introduced into the tubal ampulla confirmed diagnosis of the *Chlamydia trachomatis* infection.

Fig. 5.2.7a & b Pelvic inflammatory disease.
a Perihepatic adhesions occurring in a patient with suspected pelvic inflammatory disease.

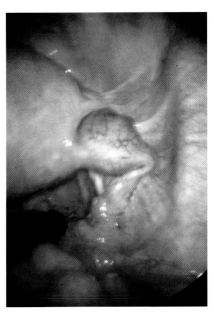

Fig. 5.2.8a & b Right isthmic tubal pregnancy.
a The isthmus is displayed showing the distension caused by the tubal pregnancy.

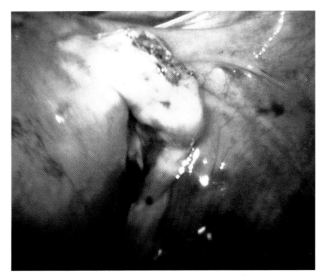

b Linear salpingotomy and evacuation of the pregnancy. The extreme blanching is due to vasopressin.

Ectopic Pregnancy

Endoscopic surgery for ectopic pregnancy is only feasible when the conceptus is in the fallopian tube. Cornual pregnancy and pregnancy in the proximal isthmus require incision of the uterine horn. Because of its vascularity and the need to close the defect, removal of these pregnancies is beyond the scope of endoscopic intervention.

When future fertility is not important, salpingectomy may be performed, but when conservative treatment is planned there is a choice between linear salpingotomy and partial resection of the tube.

First blood and clots are removed and adhesiolysis is performed to improve access. Vasopressin should be injected into the mesosalpinx at the proximal border of

the tubal dilatation to reduce bleeding. The haematosalpinx is then incised on its proximal side in an avascular zone. There has been controversy regarding the optimal site of the incision but, in practice, the anatomy is usually so distorted that the incision must be made where the haematoma reaches the surface of the tube regardless of whether it is on the mesenteric or antimesenteric border. The products are then evacuated by suction and rinsing (Fig. 5.2.8). This is usually easier when there is a large haematoma as pregnancies which cause only minor distortion of the tube are probably better anchored to the tubal wall. Haemostasis must be completed using bipolar coagulation, taking special care if vasopressin has been used and, finally, pelvic lavage is performed.

In isthmic implantation, segmental salpingectomy may be preferable. Following pelvic lavage, the tube is coagulated proximally and distally to the conceptus, and divided and removed after coagulating the mesosalpinx. Vasopressin is of less benefit in these cases and haemostasis must be achieved with coagulation, or rarely by suturing.

Adnexal Torsion

Torsion of the ovary, fallopian tube or a hydatid cyst is a common cause of acute pelvic pain. The possibility of ovarian malignancy should always be considered and ultrasonography performed prior to operative intervention. Any ovarian mass, other than simple unilocular cysts, should be treated by laparotomy.

Torsion of a hydatid cyst is treated simply by aspiration of the cyst and removal. If the tube or ovary is involved, thrombosis prophylaxis with 5000–10,000 units of heparin given slowly intravenously is recommended prior to surgical reduction of the torsion. Next the cyst or hydrosalpinx is aspirated. The torsion is then reduced and the organs are returned to their normal anatomical positions. If there is a possibility that the torsion will recur, usually because the ovarian ligament is abnormally long, the ligament is shortened by a suture ligature or a ligature around a kink in the ligament. The former method may possibly interfere less with the vascular supply to the ligament, but the loop ligature is easier to apply.

Conclusion

Laparoscopy gives access to the pelvic cavity with inherent operative risks comparable to those of laparotomy but with less postoperative morbidity. It should be considered not only as a diagnostic tool but as a procedure which permits both diagnosis and treatment, with minimal inconvenience to the patient and with results which, in some cases, may be superior to those of conventional surgery.

5.3 LASER LAPAROSCOPY

Dan C. Martin

The use of laser has become popular over the past 20 years because it allows precise tissue destruction with instruments whose effect is highly predictable.

In gynaecology, carbon dioxide (CO_2) laser was first used to treat cervical erosions and later for malignant disease and reconstructive tubal surgery. Improved prism and lens systems have since led to the application of laser to intraperitoneal tissue using CO_2 laser through the laparoscope. This had disadvantages because until recently it was transmitted through a rigid lens system. However, lasers such as argon, neodymium:yttrium-aluminium-garnet (Nd:YAG) laser, Nd:YAG laser with sapphire tips, and 532 nm potassium-titanyl-phosphate (KTP) laser, use fibre transmission and are therefore more versatile. The type of laser and delivery system chosen depends upon the exact tissue reaction desired (Fig. 5.3.1). Also the power and type of delivery system influence the effect of the laser energy.

Physical Characteristics of Laser

When CO_2 laser at high power density is applied to a tissue, the thermal damage usually extends to a depth of 0.2–0.4 mm. However, at lower power densities, the thermal effect spreads resulting in coagulation extending to a depth of 0.4–2.7 mm. Using lens systems to transmit the laser, it is possible in theory to focus the beam to a spot size as small as 0.1 mm creating a very high power density. These small spot sizes can rarely be maintained however and the effect of the power density is better understood in terms of an impact area in the depth of field (Fig. 5.3.2). Moreover, when the laser is transmitted with a laparoscope, it reflects from the side walls of the laser channel, increasing both the impact spot size and the depth of field; this can decrease the power density by as much as 52%.

In contrast to CO_2 laser, argon and KTP lasers have an intrinsic depth of penetration of 0.4–0.8 mm, whereas Nd:YAG laser penetrates 0.3–4.2 mm depending on the delivery system. However, the beam from a fibre spreads out from the maximal power density at the tip of the fibre to increasingly lower power density in the periphery (Fig. 5.3.3). Vaporization occurs only in the immediate vicinity of the fibre tip and coagulation in a zone surrounding this, but as the distance increases to about 2 cm however, the thermal effect is lost.

Small spot sizes of 0.2–0.8 mm can create high power densities of greater than 4750 watts/cm^2 and are used for clean incision and excision of tissues. Larger spot sizes of 1–3 mm produce a more haemostatic incision which is useful on the cervix and for fibromyomata. However, these low power densities of 400–4000 watts/cm^2 also result in dessication, increased carbonization and increased smoke production. High power densities can be controlled with the use of superpulse, repeat pulse or a combination of the two. These techniques increase the control of high power density by lowering the average power density.

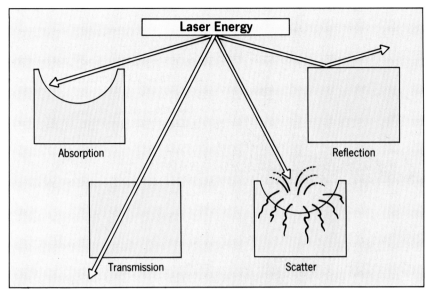

Fig. 5.3.1a & b Lasers.

a Laser energy is transmitted, reflected, absorbed or scattered. Absorption results in heating, coagulation, burning or vaporization Vaporization is the most useful effect with the CO_2 laser.

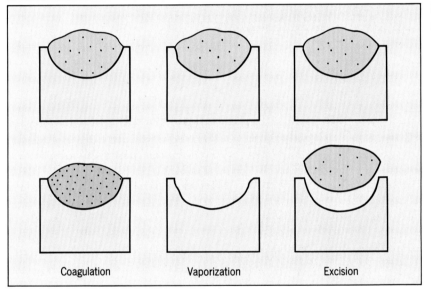

b Lasers can be controlled to produce coagulation, vaporization and excision.

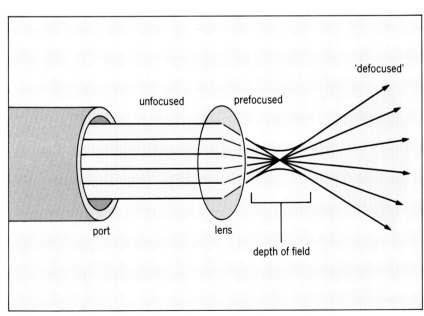

Fig. 5.3.2 A laser exits from its port and is focused by a lens.
Depending on the lens characteristics and focal length, the system has a depth of field in which the spot size and power density remains relatively constant.

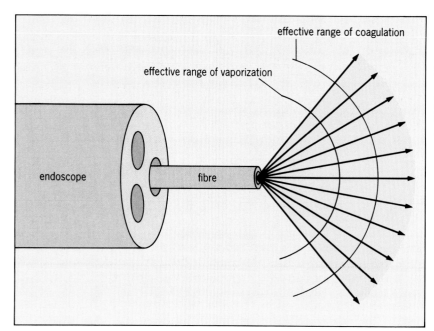

Fig. 5.3.3 As the laser beam exits from a fibre, it diverges rapidly.
At high power density, vaporization is possible in the area near the tip of the fibre. Past this, coagulation occurs. At far distances (i.e. greater than 1–2 cm), the power density has decreased below the threshold of coagulation.

Tubal Reconstructive Surgery

The first intra-abdominal gynaecological use of laser was in tubal reconstructive surgery. Attempts to use the heat production of laser to weld tissues have been unsuccessful, but the use of pulse and superpulse modes have decreased tubal damage and lessened the incidence of tubal stenosis. Although hand-held instruments can produce peak power densities of up to 45,000 watts/cm^2, they should be avoided as they also produce low power density that can cause tubal stenosis.

Some microsurgeons have concluded that tubal anastomosis can be performed with laser more rapidly, more easily and with better haemostasis than with conventional methods. In contrast, others have noted no increase in the success rates, but have reported a higher risk of tubal stenosis and inadvertent thermal damage unless power densities are maintained at greater than 4750–20,000 watts/cm^2. Thus most microsurgeons have found that conventional techniques are better than laser for tubal anastomosis. However, the use of laser for cuff salpingostomy has decreased the operating time, and led to increased haemostasis, thus increasing the use of laparoscopy for this procedure.

Endometriosis

Endometriosis is the most common indication for the use of laser laparoscopy. Suppression of endometrial activity by medical treatment has decreased pain and increased pregnancy rates, but recurrence of clinical disease after cessation of treatment is common. Complete surgical excision and destruction of endometriosis is, however, more successful in treating pain and in preventing long-term recurrence or persistence of the disease.

Although destruction or excision is limited to visible and predictable disease, microlaparoscopy can be used to see small and subtle lesions. CO_2 laser can be used to vaporize or excise these lesions, whereas argon, Nd:YAG and KTP lasers can be used to coagulate or vaporize them.

Previously ablation tended to increase carbonization, obscuring the appearance of endometriosis both during the surgical procedure and, later, at second-look laparoscopy. Excision of these carbon areas showed that they were associated with a foreign body giant cell reaction. Therefore, lavage and pusher sponges should be used to remove excess carbon and improve visibility which is impaired due to tissue distortion.

Small Peritoneal Lesions

Laser therapy of small lesions is easier by vaporization and coagulation than by excision, but vaporization of larger lesions leads to excessive smoke production. When vaporization is being performed, it must be taken down to healthy tissue. During excision of lesions, the perimeter is first vaporized to form a cut edge and then the lesion is lifted forwards to facilitate excision of its base. In addition, biopsies must be obtained for histological confirmation if there is doubt about the diagnosis of endometriosis.

Blunt dissection of deep tissue is used in many situations. Preservation of the ureter is one of the most important of these, and it is safer to separate it from the lateral peritoneum by blunt dissection to ensure that the laser is never aimed directly at it.

Deep lesions in the pouch of Douglas can be excised by a combination of laser laparoscopy and posterior colpotomy. They are first dissected by laser as far as the vaginal fascia and then colpotomy is performed under laparoscopic control. These deep lesions can then be removed through the vaginal incision which is closed at the completion of the operation.

Nodules which can be felt in the pouch of Douglas may not be visible laparoscopically, therefore a rectal examination should be performed after the excision to ensure that the removal has been complete.

If the patient has been experiencing pain and if nodularity is still present, the dissection is continued either laparoscopically (Fig. 5.3.4) or via a vaginal approach. On the other hand, if the indication for surgery is infertility and pain is not a factor, any residual nodules may be treated medically or even expectantly.

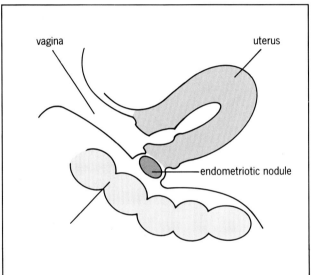

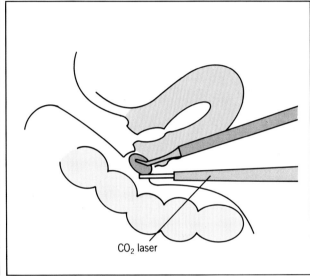

Fig. 5.3.4a–d Resection of endometriosis in the pouch of Douglas.
a Nodule of endometriosis in the recto-vaginal septum.

b CO$_2$ laser is used to dissect the peritoneal aspect of the nodule.

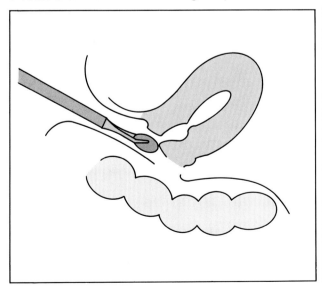

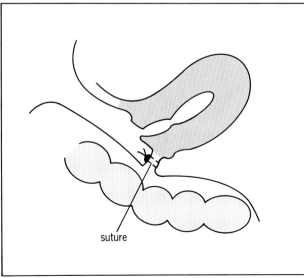

c Posterior colpotomy allows complete removal.

d The colpotomy incision is closed.

Ovarian Endometriosis

The treatment of ovarian endometriosis is preferably performed by high power density beams which give a better control over the depth to which these areas are vaporized, than that possible with low power density. Endometriotic lesions of less than 5 mm in diameter should be biopsied and the base ablated with laser. Vaporization is then continued until normal white ovarian tissue appears. Histological examination of the residual adherent ovary often shows that the endometriosis extended more deeply than was originally appreciated.

Larger endometriomata of 2–5 cm diameter are best enucleated. They are first opened by laser, irrigated and examined (Fig. 5.3.5). The edge of the wall of the endometrioma is then teased out and stripped as in pelviscopy. In order to locate the correct tissue plane for dissection, the endometrioma should be opened at its most dependant point by grasping the opened edge and using the laser to make a relieving incision whilst the edge is held under tension. The correct tissue plane then becomes apparent whilst the relieving incision helps to prevent tearing and bleeding of the proximal ovarian margin. Histological examination of large endometriomata will demonstrate flattening of the endometriosis on the internal lining wall.

Laser treatment of endometriomata which exceed 5 cm in diameter is technically difficult; the tissue planes are not easy to recognize and the procedure can take several hours to perform. The ovarian shell collapses during the operation making complete resection difficult to guarantee.

Ovarian endometriomata are frequently adherent to the broad ligament. In this situation, the broad ligament must be excised as it is frequently infiltrated with endometriosis which cannot be seen through the adhesions.

Postoperative Adhesion Formation

Adhesion formation following laser laparoscopy has not presented a problem clinically or in laboratory studies. Adhesions are more likely to be caused by ischaemia associated with suturing, whereas the necrotic tissue resulting from the use of laser, bipolar or thermal coagulation does not seem to produce signficant adhesion formation (Semm, 1982). However, adhesion reformation continues to be of concern and appears to be related more to the disease or to the patient than to the technique used.

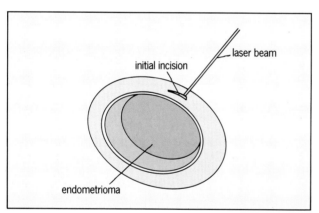

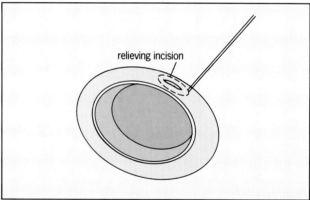

Fig. 5.3.5a–d Resection of ovarian endometriosis.
a An incision is made in the wall of the endometrioma with laser.

b A relieving incision is made through healthy ovarian tissue around the endometrioma.

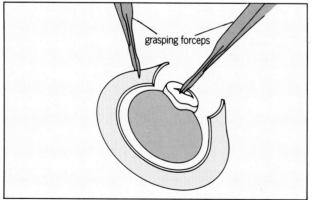

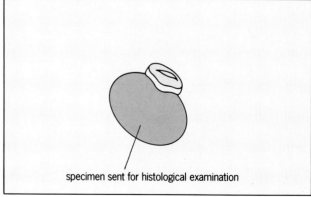

c The endometrioma is stripped out of the ovary by traction with forceps.

d The endometrioma is submitted for histological examination.

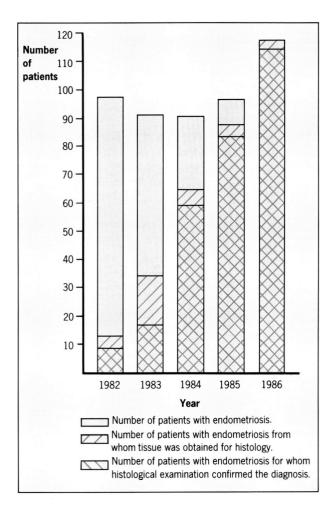

Number of patients with endometriosis.

Number of patients with endometriosis from whom tissue was obtained for histology.

Number of patients with endometriosis for whom histological examination confirmed the diagnosis.

Advantages

Laser excision produces excellent tissue for histological confirmation of the diagnosis of endometriosis and the improved techniques have increased confirmation of the diagnosis from 62% in 1982 to 97% in 1986 (Martin & Vander Zwaag, 1987) (Fig. 5.3.6).Thus, awareness of the extent and variety of the presentations of peritoneal and ovarian endometriosis has increased (Martin, 1986).

Fertility following laser surgery for endometriosis is good and reproducible (Fig. 5.3.7) whether CO_2 or argon laser is used. Life table analysis has demonstrated that the use of CO_2 laser laparoscopy in both mild and moderate endometriosis produces equally good, yet more rapid, results than laparotomy or medical suppression. Furthermore, in severe endometriosis, the success rate is equal to or greater than that of laparotomy or medical treatment (Martin & Diamond, 1986).

When pain is the indication for surgery, the CO_2 laser allows the dissection to extend more deeply into the pelvis than with previous techniques. This has resulted in better recognition and more complete removal of the lesions and, in the short term, improved pain relief and a decreased need for a repeat operation.

Fig. 5.3.6 Confirming the diagnosis of endometriosis.
With the increasing use of laser excision for obtaining tissue, confirmation of the diagnosis of endometriosis has increased. (From Martin & Vander Zwaag, 1987.)

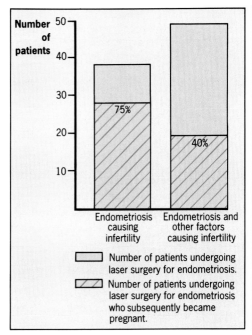

Number of patients undergoing laser surgery for endometriosis.

Number of patients undergoing laser surgery for endometriosis who subsequently became pregnant.

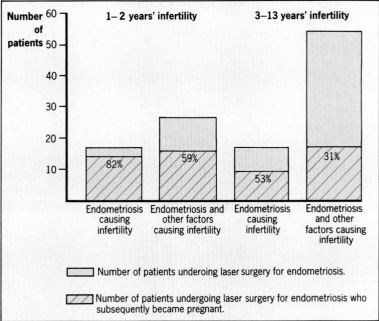

Number of patients undergoing laser surgery for endometriosis.

Number of patients undergoing laser surgery for endometriosis who subsequently became pregnant.

Fig. 5.3.7 a & b Laser surgery for endometriosis.
a Fertility after laser surgery for endometriosis is good if endometriosis is the only factor causing infertility. (From Martin & Diamond, 1986.)

b Pregnancy rates following laser surgery for endometriosis depend on the number of years of infertility at the time of surgery and the presence of other factors causing infertility. (From Martin, 1986.)

Ectopic Pregnancy

The treatment of ectopic pregnancy may be salpingectomy, conservative surgery or medical management with methotrexate. Linear salpingostomy (Fig. 5.3.8a) has been performed with CO_2 laser, argon laser and KTP laser. These procedures are of most value when the ectopic pregnancy is diagnosed in the first 22–27 days. After this time, salpingectomy becomes increasingly useful. When using the CO_2 laser, button-type coagulator irrigators are useful for focal coagulation of bleeding from the base of the ectopic implantation. Vasopressin injection also helps to decrease this bleeding.

After conservative surgery for ectopic pregnancy, viable trophoblastic material may persist whether the operation has been performed by laparotomy or laparoscopy. If tubal conservation is not necessary, as when salpingoscopy shows evidence of focal mucosal damage, laparoscopic salpingectomy with coagulation and scissors is easier than salpingostomy (Fig. 5.3.8b).

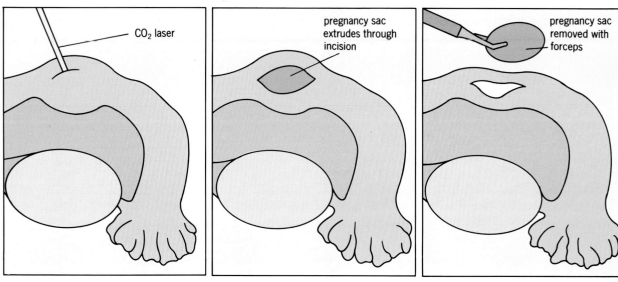

Fig. 5.3.8a & b The use of laser in the surgical treatment of ectopic pregnancy.
Ectopic pregnancy is treated by salpingostomy and salpingectomy.
a Linear salpingostomy for an ampullary ectopic pregnancy is performed with the use of the laser beam to open the tube. The products of conception are grasped and removed. The incision is allowed to heal without primary closure.

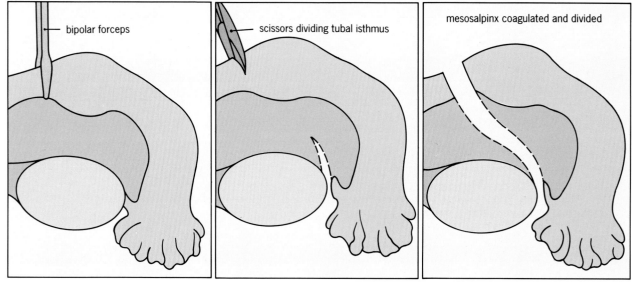

b Salpingectomy is performed using bipolar coagulation and scissors.

Adhesiolysis

Higher power densities of 3000–20,000 watts/cm^2 are used with CO_2 laser to incise adhesions, but a backstop and barriers are needed for limiting its penetration (Fig. 5.3.9). Argon, KTP and Nd:YAG lasers have been used as well, but their depth of penetration is limited by divergence of the beam and backstops are less important.

The use of lasers for dissecting tubal and ovarian adhesions decreases the risk of inadvertent damage from thermal or electrical coagulators. Fig. 5.3.10a shows a tube that is densely adherent to the uterus and ovary, and Fig. 5.3.10b shows it being freed from the uterine fundus by the laser used in a high power density mode. The adhesions are then removed from the ovary, and the dense adhesions between the ovary and the uterus are resected (Figs 5.3.10c & d). Finally, any excess carbon is brushed from the excisional site leaving clean incisional fields (Figs 5.3.10e & f).

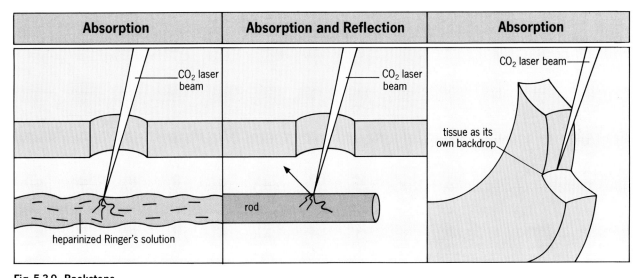

Fig. 5.3.9 Backstops.
Backstops are used to limit the penetration of the CO_2 laser. Solutions are the easiest to use and absorb the energy. Rods both absorb and reflect the energy. In some cases, such as opening a hydrosalpinx, the tissue can serve as its own backstop.

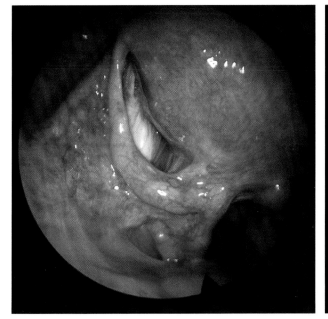

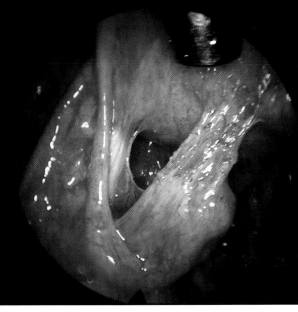

Fig. 5.3.10a–f Laser dissection of adhesions.
a The tube is densely adherent to the uterus and ovary.

b The laser is used in the high power density mode to free the tube from the uterine fundus.

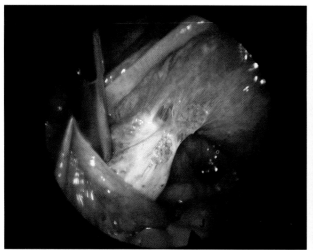

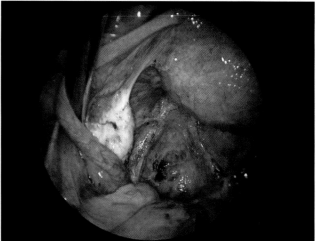

Fig. 5.3.10 continued.

c The ovarian adhesions are then lysed.

d All adhesions have been lysed and resected.

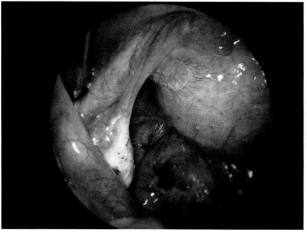

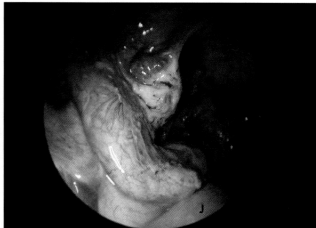

e Excess carbon is brushed from the ovarian site.

f Excess carbon has been brushed from the tubal site.

Cuff Salpingostomy

Intrauterine pregnancy rates of 25–30% have been reported following laparoscopic cuff salpingostomy with the CO_2 laser (Taylor *et al.*, 1986). The wall of the hydrosalpinx is incised radially and longitudinally by laser (Fig. 5.3.11a), and the serosal edge is everted using a low power density beam of 50–200 watts/cm^2 to coagulate the serosa and turn back the edge (Fig. 5.3.11b–d). At the end of the procedure, the walls are held apart by the coagulated and contracted serosa (Fig. 5.3.11e). The degree of eversion should be exaggerated because early cases were complicated by closure due to insufficient coagulation. The coagulation can be carried to a point where vaporization of the serosa occurs, as second-look laparoscopy indicates that this does not cause adhesions. Argon and KTP lasers have also been used to carry out this procedure. The resultant pregnancy rate shows a greater relationship with the state of the mucosal folds than with the technique used.

Reversal of Sterilization

Tubal anastomoses have been performed laparoscopically using the endocoagulator, electrosurgical techniques and CO_2 laser. No viable or ongoing pregnancies

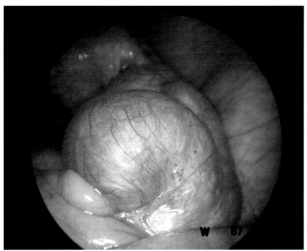

Fig. 5.3.11a–e Laparoscopic cuff salpingostomy with laser.
a The wall of a hydrosalpinx is incised longitudinally and radially using the CO_2 laser.

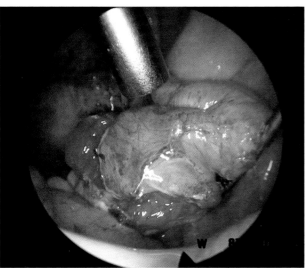

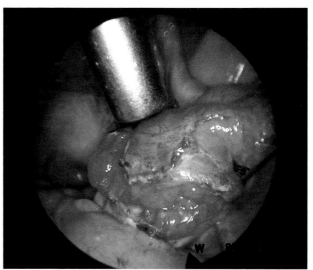

b The low power density mode of the beam is aimed at the serosal surface of the tube to cause a surface coagulation.

c As coagulation begins, the edges evert.

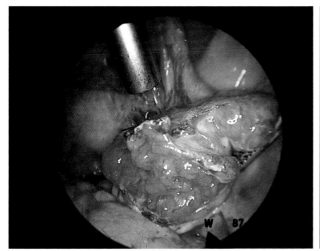

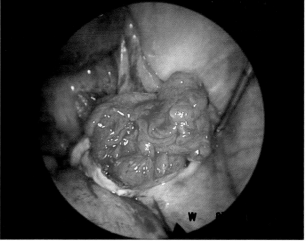

d With continued coagulation, the edges continue to retract and the endosalpinx is seen.

e At the end of the procedure, the walls are held apart by the coagulated and contracted serosa. This eversion should be exaggerated as early cases were complicated by closure due to insufficient separation of the edges.

have been reported but three miscarriages and two tubal pregnancies have occurred. In contrast, mini-laparotomy and microsurgical anastomoses have been performed as an outpatient procedure with the accompanying success rates of microsurgery and the financial savings of outpatient surgery.

Complications

The complications of laparoscopy and laser laparoscopy (Fig. 5.3.12) are identical though the latter carries the added risks of the extent of surgery. Laser laparoscopy increases surgical precision and avoids the need for laparotomy in many cases. The author reports only one emergency laparotomy in his first 702 cases.

Safety

Safety must be a major concern in the use of laparoscopic equipment. It is important that the following guidelines are met.
1. The patient must not be put at unnecessary risk.

2. The indications for this type of surgery are not increased inappropriately.
3. The surgeon recognizes the limitations of his own skill. This applies particularly to the use of new instruments and techniques as it may take months or years to acquire the new skills and, indeed, the better the surgeon is with older techniques, the harder it is to change to new methods. Surgeons wishing to develop these new techniques should attend one of the courses available in many countries as well as familiarize themselves with the physical properties of laser and the safety manuals in its use.

Conclusion

Laser laparoscopy is part of the larger body of operative laparoscopy. Lasers, bipolar coagulators, thermal coagulators, sharp incision and unipolar knives have different tissue effects and the choice of instrument used will depend on the effect desired as well as the skill of the operator. Continued study is necessary to clarify the most appropriate equipment for a given operative procedure.

Complications of Laparoscopy	Complications of Operative Laparoscopy
Hypothermia	Complications of laparoscopy
Haemorrhage requiring blood transfusion	+
Cardiac arrest	Loss of pusher sponge
Dissecting emphysema	Haemorrhage from deep pelvic vessels
Laparotomy	Partial amputation of hydrosalpinx
Laceration of major vessels	Transection of fallopian tube
Bowel damage	Incision of bowel by laser
	Incision of ureter by laser

Fig. 5.3.12 Complications of laparoscopy and operative laparoscopy.

5.4 NEW TECHNIQUES OF TUBAL GAMETE AND EMBRYO TRANSFER
Ricardo H. Asch and Rita Guidetti

Introduction

It is generally accepted that fertilization of the human oöcyte by sperm and early embryonic development takes place in the lumen of the fallopian tube at the junction of the ampulla and isthmus. The fertilized ovum remains at the ampullary-isthmic junction for about 80 hours, undergoing cleavage to reach the 16–32 blastomere stage before entering the uterus where it develops into a full blastocyst.

If infertility is caused by disease or obstruction of the fallopian tubes, *in vitro* fertilization and embryo transfer (IVF–ET) is the only treatment currently available if surgical correction of the abnormal tubes is not possible. Although IVF–ET was originally designed as a therapy for women with severely damaged or absent fallopian tubes, in recent years it has also been proposed and used to overcome infertility due to other causes in whom traditional or conventional infertility therapy has failed. A number of these women have anatomically intact tubes which are theoretically capable of normal gamete transport and of presenting a favourable milieu for early embryonic development. In these women the alleged embryotrophic properties of the tube are not used when *in vitro* fertilization involves the transfer of the embryos through the cervix into the uterus.

Studies on rhesus monkeys showed that the transfer of embryos to the uterus is followed by a lower rate of pregnancy and a higher rate of abortion than when embryos are transferred into the fallopian tubes. Similar experiments on mice and sheep have shown that tubal epithelial factors are important both in producing optimal embryonic growth in culture and in enabling transferred embryos to survive beyond the stage of implantation. Thus, in 1984, gamete intrafallopian transfer (GIFT) was developed as a form of therapy for infertile women with at least one anatomically and functionally intact fallopian tube (Asch *et al.*, 1985). The main theoretical advantage of this method lies in the assumption that fertilization of the oöcyte and early development takes place as in spontaneous human conception, in the ampullary-isthmic junction of the fallopian tube, overcoming any defects in tubal transport. GIFT ensures that microscopically normal oöcytes and motile spermatozoa reach the normal site of fertilization, and increases the chance of implantation.

A new technique, tubal embryo transfer (TET) – also known as zygote intrafallopian transfer (ZIFT) or pronuclear stage tubal transfer (PROST) – has been proposed by several authors, with the idea of combining the advantages of both IVF and GIFT (Yovich *et al.*, 1987; Devroey *et al.*, 1986). The introduction of an ultrasound guided technique for follicular aspiration permits oöcyte retrieval without the need for a major surgical intervention, therefore the embryos generated after IVF can be transferred into the fallopian tubes by performing only one surgical procedure. TET combines the advantages of IVF (i.e. a controlled fertilization), with those of GIFT (i.e. the provision of a more physiological pre-implantation development and transport of the embryos). However, both GIFT and TET currently involve gamete or embryo transfer by laparoscopy under general anaesthesia. This need for surgery limits repetitive attempts to improve the chance of pregnancy and significantly increases the cost of each attempt.

Recently, a non-surgical tubal embryo or gamete transfer via the cervix has been proposed as an alternative that obviates the need for an invasive approach.

Gamete Intrafallopian Transfer (GIFT)

Gamete intrafallopian transfer (GIFT) involves the direct transfer of preovulatory oöcytes and washed sperm into the fallopian tubes, and has been found to be a successful treatment for infertile women with at least one normal tube; subsequent pregnancy rates have been higher than those after IVF and the risk of spontaneous abortion has been lower.

Originally GIFT was proposed for women with unexplained infertility, but the indications have since been extended to include conditions such as mild to moderate endometriosis, male infertility, failure of several cycles of artificial insemination with husband's or donor sperm, cervical stenosis and cases of premature ovarian failure using donor oöcytes.

Preparation of the Female Partner
Before undergoing GIFT, tubal patency and normal tubal morphology must be proved either by laparoscopy or hysterosalpingography (HSG).

In a GIFT cycle, controlled ovarian hyperstimulation is followed by retrieval, examination and incubation of the oöcytes, which are then mixed with sperm and transferred into the fallopian tubes (Fig. 5.4.1).

Controlled ovarian hyperstimulation is induced using a combination of clomiphene citrate, gonadotrophin releasing hormone analogues (GnRH), follicle stimulating hormone (FSH) and human menopausal gonadotrophin (HMG). Follicular development is monitored by ultrasound, and human chorionic gonadotrophin (HCG) is administered when at least two or three follicles reach a mean diameter of 16–17 mm and the level of serum oestradiol is greater than 250 pg/ml per follicle.

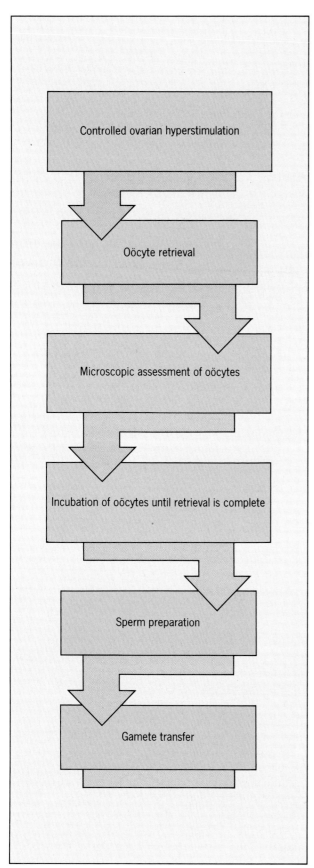

Fig. 5.4.1 Chronology of a GIFT cycle.

Oöcyte retrieval can be performed by laparoscopy or by vaginal aspiration under ultrasound control approximately 35 hours after the injection of HCG. The retrieved oöcytes are classified as type 0 to type 5; type 0 are degenerate and atretic, whereas type 5 are preovulatory with a radiating cumulus corona complex and a visible polar body. The most mature oöcytes are selected and loaded into a catheter with an appropriate number of sperm (100,000–500,000 in 25 μl), and two oöcytes are transferred into each tube. If there is a severe male factor, more oöcytes and sperm may be transferred.

Preparation of the Sperm
Prior to undertaking assisted fertilization, at least two semen analyses are performed, together with antibody testing and bacteriological culture. On the day of the GIFT, the sperm is prepared by wash and swim-up, Percoll or sedimentation techniques. If there is oligospermia, a semen sample may be stored in an egg yolk buffer medium at 2–5°C for 48 hours. With this approach an extra sample of sperm is available and, at the same time, the sperm capacitation process is enhanced.

Results of GIFT
The clinical pregnancy rate with GIFT ranges from 32–34% (Fig. 5.4.2), but the results are lower when a male factor is present although the success is variable (Fig. 5.4.3). Despite WHO parameters for classifying a semen sample as normal, there are no conventional seminal parameters that might have a predictive value on the oöcyte fertilization or pregnancy rate in oligoasthenospermic men. Our criteria are shown in Fig. 5.4.4; if these are fulfilled, GIFT is offered, otherwise TET is the chosen method of treatment.

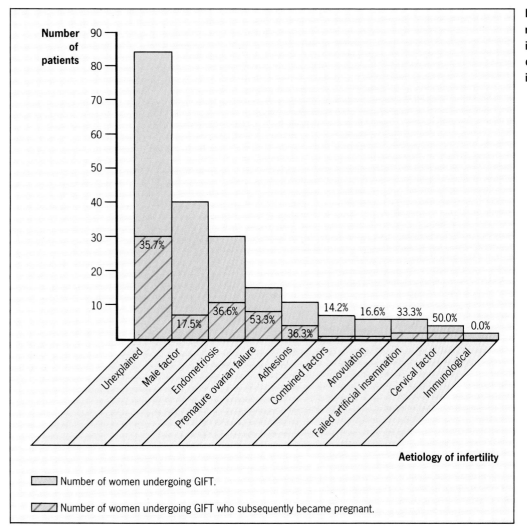

Fig. 5.4.2 Pregnancy rates following GIFT in women with different causes of infertility.

Study	Number of cases	Resulting pregnancies	
		Number	%
Multicentre group study (1987, Australia and New Zealand)	397	61	15
Matson *et al.* (1987, Australia)	32	6	18
Leeton *et al.* (1987, Australia)	6	2	33
Wong *et al.* (1986, Singapore)	18	3	16
Nishi (Japan)	32	13	40
Cittadini (Italy)	37	9	24
Rolet (France)	14	0	0
Borrero *et al.* (1988, USA)	30	4	13

Fig. 5.4.3 Pregnancy rates following GIFT for male infertility.

WHO standards

Higher sperm count with progression of 1 before treatment

Higher sperm count with progression of 1–2 after treatment

Sperm morphology with <25% normal forms

Repetitive failure of fertilization of human oöcytes *in vitro*

Failure of fertilization in two or more Hamster Tests

Fig. 5.4.4 Criteria for defining male factor infertility.

Tubal Embryo Transfer (TET)

Experience gained from the GIFT programme has shown that the results for couples with severe male factor infertility are significantly lower than for couples with other causes of infertility, for example unexplained infertility, endometriosis, cervical factor, failed donor insemination and oöcyte donation for premature ovarian failure.

Experimental research in a non-human primate model indicated that normal intra-uterine pregnancies could be achieved after transferring embryos resulting from IVF into the fallopian tube. The application of a similar technique in a clinical situation has proved successful for specific causes of infertility. This procedure has been called zygote intrafallopian transfer (ZIFT), pronuclear stage tubal transfer (PROST) or tubal embryo transfer (TET).

In TET, the oöcytes are recovered by transvaginal ultrasound and incubated in the laboratory with prepared sperms according to conventional IVF technique. Tubal transfer is performed by laparoscopy 24–52 hours later, and the resultant pregnancy rate is approximately 28% per cycle and 45% per transfer. To assess the efficiency of TET, the results must be compared to those of other treatment procedures and, although the figures are still small, the results are encouraging in male factor infertility (Fig. 5.4.5) compared to those following GIFT (17%) or IVF (10%). Moreover, the incidence of ectopic pregnancy does not appear to be higher than with IVF or GIFT.

This combination of IVF and GIFT technology has been considered acceptable because it offers the advantages of confirming the occurrence of fertilization, exposing the very early embryo to the natural tubal environment, and allowing the uterine environment to become less hostile. Moreover, in contrast to GIFT, the patient is not subjected to surgery unless there is laboratory confirmation of fertilization.

Non-Surgical Gamete or Embryo Tubal Transfer

When performed by laparoscopy or minilaparotomy, tubal gamete (GIFT) or embryo (TET) transfers are surgical procedures requiring general anaesthesia and

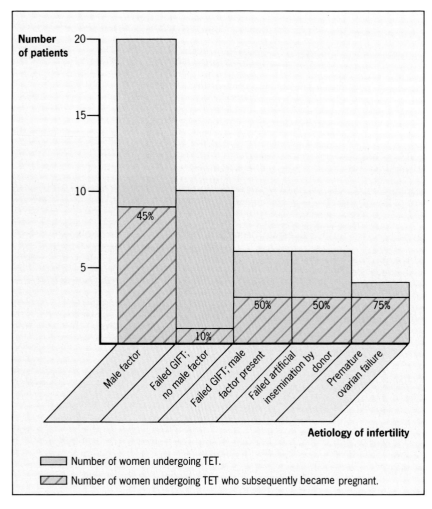

Fig. 5.4.5 Pregnancy rates following TET for certain specific causes of infertility.
Based on data from the UCI Center for Reproductive Health, January–June 1988.

hospitalization. The need for surgery constitutes a serious limitation in the decision to repeat these procedures on multiple occasions in order to improve the chances of pregnancy, and also significantly increases the cost of each attempt. Non-surgical intratubal gamete or embryo transfer has recently been proposed as an alternative (Jansen & Anderson, 1987), and ultrasound guided embryo transfer into the fallopian tube via the cervix by Jansen *et al.* (1988), has resulted in pregnancies. Bustillo *et al.* (1988) have also reported a pregnancy resulting from GIFT after non-surgical ultrasound guided selective tubal catheterization. The instruments used consist of a malleable obturator in a 5.5 F uterine teflon sheath which is pre-curved and its memory directs it towards the utero-tubal junction when the obturator is removed. When the sheath is confirmed by ultrasound to be pointing towards the tubal ostium, a 3 F teflon catheter tapered to 2 F at the tip is advanced into the fallopian tube 3 cm beyond the sheath tip, and the gametes or embryos are injected. Other catheters with a platinum tip, which is radio-opaque, may be used. A hysteroscopic approach has also been advocated either for the recanalization of a proximally blocked tube or for embryo or gamete transfer, with encouraging early results.

Although these techniques appear to be safe and relatively easy office procedures, significant limitations still exist which prevent their widespread application.

The ultrasound non-surgical tubal cannulation technique is effective in approximately 68% of all subjects. To improve these rates, more reliable devices have to be developed. As well as difficulties visualizing the catheter by ultrasound, the volume of fluid injected into the tube has not yet been well established, and it is not yet known if the contractility of the proximal tube can be affected by the volume of fluid used. Further, it is still not clear whether repeated tubal catheterization via the utero-tubal ostium could be traumatic.

At present GIFT or TET via laparoscopy is still preferred to the use of non-surgical techniques. However, development and improvement of non-surgical techniques may provide a more attractive alternative method of gamete or embryo transfer for the treatment of non-tubal infertility in the future.

5.5 EPILOGUE

The introduction of new, efficient methods for the surgical treatment of female infertility has dramatically changed the prognosis for women with this distressing condition.

Tubal disease resulting from pelvic infection or endometriosis is the most common cause of long-standing infertility. Whilst microsurgical techniques have proved to be highly successful in reversal of sterilization, they are less effective for women with pathological proximal tubal obstruction, and are only marginally better than conventional surgery for the treatment of occlusion of the distal end of the fallopian tube (Fig. 5.5.1). However, in women with hydrosalpinx, when preliminary salpingoscopy has demonstrated a normal ampullary mucosa, microsurgery can offer a pregnancy rate of more than 50% (De Bruyne *et al.*, 1989), and similar results have been obtained with both conventional and laser laparoscopic surgery.

The advent of *in vitro* fertilization has altered the outlook for women with tubal mucosal damage or inoperable tubal obstruction. These women, who were previously sterile, may now be offered a chance of pregnancy which varies between 10–20% per ovum recovery procedure. Laparoscopic ovum retrieval has been complemented in most centres by an ultrasound directed transvaginal approach. This less invasive procedure has facilitated the development of tubal embryo transfer and made possible new non-operative techniques for assisted fertilization. The correct selection of cases for treatment by surgery, *in vitro* fertilization, tubal gamete or zygote transfer remains a most important aspect in the management of the woman with tubal infertility. The success of gamete intrafallopian transfer and tubal embryo transfer are both based on the normal morphology and function of the fallopian tubes. However, either technique may be complicated by ectopic pregnancy so it is important that the tube is fully evaluated prior to treatment in order to avoid this potentially serious complication.

Endometriosis is also a disease where the clinician is faced with major diagnostic and therapeutic problems. We still do not have a complete understanding of its pathophysiology and, therefore, assessment of the results of treatment remains difficult. Mild endometriosis may be treated medically, surgically or expectantly, with a similar degree of success. However moderate and severe endometriosis should be treated surgically, but the results in terms of fecundity are similar whether conventional microsurgery or laparoscopic surgery are used (Olive & Haney, 1986).

Postoperative adhesion formation is a risk of any reconstructive pelvic surgery. Before proposing a rational approach to the prevention and treatment of adhesions, the factors determining the progress of the disease and the mechanism of its association with infertility need to be elucidated, and the optimum therapy determined by controlled prospective studies.

This book has been written to contribute in a small way to the understanding of these important causes of infertility.

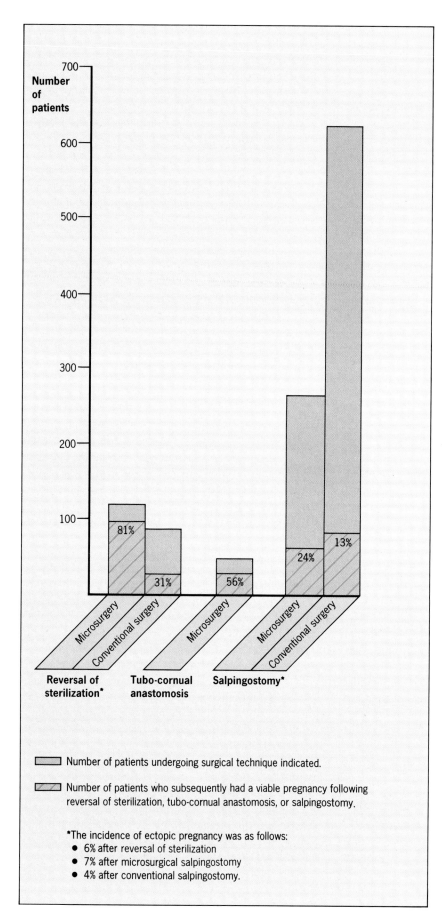

Fig. 5.5.1 Success of microsurgical techniques in reversal of sterilization and for pathological proximal tubal obstruction.
Based on data of Gomel (1983) and Soules (1986).

Number of patients undergoing surgical technique indicated.

Number of patients who subsequently had a viable pregnancy following reversal of sterilization, tubo-cornual anastomosis, or salpingostomy.

*The incidence of ectopic pregnancy was as follows:
- 6% after reversal of sterilization
- 7% after microsurgical salpingostomy
- 4% after conventional salpingostomy.

REFERENCES

Asch, R.H., Balmaceda, J.P., Ellsworth, L.R. & Wong, P.C. (1985) Gamete intrafallopian transfer (GIFT): a new treatment for infertility. *International Journal of Fertility*, **30**, 41–45.

Bustillo, M., Munabi, A.K. & Schulman, J.D. (1988) Pregnancy after nonsurgical ultrasound-guided gamete intrafallopian transfer. *New England Journal of Medicine*, **319**, 313.

Cherney, L.S. (1941) A modified transverse incision for low abdominal operations. *Surgery, Gynecology and Obstetrics*, **72**, 92–95.

Devroey, P., Braeckmans, P., Smitz, J. *et al.* (1986) Pregnancy after translaparoscopic zygote intrafallopian transfer in patient with sperm antibodies. *Lancet*, **1**, 1329.

De Bruyne, F., Puttemans, P., Boeckx, W. & Brosens, I. (1989) The clinical value of salpingoscopy in tubal infertility. *Fertility and Sterility*, **51**, 339–340.

Gomel, V. (1983) *Microsurgery in Female Infertility*. Boston, Toronto: Little, Brown and Company.

Jansen, R.P.S. & Anderson, J.C. (1987) Catheterization of the fallopian tubes from the vagina. *Lancet*, **2**, 309–310.

Jansen, R.P.S., Anderson, J.C. & Sutherland, P.D. (1988) Nonoperative embryo transfer to the fallopian tube. *New England Journal of Medicine*, **319**, 288–291.

Levine, R.L. (1985) Economic impact of pelviscopic surgery. *Journal of Reproductive Medicine*, **30**, 655–659.

Martin, D.C. (1986) Laser physics and practice. In *Atlas of Female Infertility Surgery*. Edited by R.B. Hunt. pp.103–111. Chicago: Yearbook Medical Publishers.

Martin, D.C. (1986) CO_2 laser laparoscopy for endometriosis associated with infertility. *Journal of Reproductive Medicine*, **31**, 1089–1094.

Martin, D.C. & Diamond, M.P. (1986) Operative laparoscopy: comparison of lasers with other techniques. *Current Problems in Obstetrics, Gynecology and Fertility*, **9(12)**, 563–601.

Martin, D.C. & Vander Zwaag, R. (1987) Excisional techniques with the CO_2 laser laparoscope. *Journal of Reproductive Medicine*, **32**, 753–758.

Olive, D.L. & Haney, A.F. (1986) Endometriosis-associated infertility: a critical review of therapeutic approaches. *Obstetrical and Gynecological Survey*, **41**, 538–555.

Palmer, R. (1974) Safety in laparoscopy. *Journal of Reproductive Medicine*, **13**, 1–5.

Rioux, J.E. (1977) *Relative Risk of Unipolar Versus Bipolar Coagulation in the Prevention and Management of Laparoscopic Complications*. Edited by J.F. Huika & C.R. Wheeless. pp.14–15. Irvine: American Association of Gynecological Laparoscopists.

Semm, K. (1982) Advances in pelviscopic surgery. *Current Problems in Obstetrics and Gynecology*, **5(10)**, 1–42.

Taylor, M.V., Martin, D.C., Poston, W., Dean, P.J. & Vander Zwaag, R. (1986) Effect of power density and carbonization on residual tissue coagulation using the continuous wave carbon dioxide laser. *Colposcopy and Gynecological Laser Surgery*, **2**, 169–175.

Soules, M.R. (1986) Infertility surgery. In *Reproductive Failure*. Edited by A.H. DeCherney. pp.117–151. Edinburgh: Churchill Livingstone.

Yovich, J.L., Matson, P.L., Blackledge, D.G., Turner, S.R., Richardson, P.A. & Draper, R. (1987) Pregnancies following pronuclear stage tubal transfer. *Fertility and Sterility*, **48**, 851–857.

INDEX